What a beautiful, holis
body, and spirit! From
techniques and moveme
practical tools and resou
mind-body connection, a... ... . reminding us of truths from Scripture
that eclipse any labels we may carry.

    JENNIFER TUCKER, author of *Breath as Prayer* and *Present in Prayer*

Live Beyond Your Label is an inspiring and insightful read that combines solid research, well-founded theory, and real-world wisdom into compelling, accessible chapters. The author's authenticity shines through, making complex ideas feel both personal and practical. This book is a valuable resource for anyone seeking to break free from limiting labels and step into their full potential with confidence and clarity.

    TAMARA ROSIER, PHD, author of *Your Brain's Not Broken*

If you're exhausted from chasing quick fixes that fail, this amazing book is full of grace, wisdom, and doable tips to help you truly heal. Throughout these pages, Erin Kerry vulnerably shares her story while offering science-backed strategies to help you pursue health in a gentle, God-honoring way. If you're tired of being talked down to or misunderstood by the medical community, read this book!

    HEATHER CREEKMORE, author of *The 40-Day Body Image Workbook* and host of the *Compared to Who?* podcast

In *Live Beyond Your Label*, author Erin Kerry unites biblical truth, functional medicine, and personal experience to offer hope and practical healing tools to those looking to change their health narrative. Erin shares her real-life journey of overcoming PTSD, depression, and bipolar disorder; and she draws from both science and Scripture to lead readers through specific ways to be well in mind, body, and spirit. This book is like meeting with your friend, health coach, and spiritual mentor all at the same time.

    CHELSEA BLACKBIRD, CHP, The Christian Nutritionist

Live Beyond Your Label breaks down the shame around mental health disorders and empowers people with the tools to heal their root issues and thrive. Erin blends science, storytelling, and supportive strategies to create a manual for health that isn't just theoretical; she and her clients are living proof that her system works.

    DR. KATE KRESGE, head of medical education, Rupa Health, a Fullscript company

Everyone in the medical community needs to read this book. Erin shares a remarkable illustration of how to heal from diseases and "labels" that many still believe are lifelong curses. We all need to take a step back, understand the dilemma that faces us, and learn how to help our patients heal from layers of trauma inflicted from both inside and outside the medical establishment. Erin beautifully blends her own story with wonderful insights that will inform even the most knowledgeable professional. Whether you are a mental health professional desiring to take a deeper look or someone seeking solutions outside of a broken health-care system, this book will offer you hope, encouragement, and ultimately wholehearted healing.

STEFANI REINOLD, MD, MPH, holistic psychiatrist, host of *The Dr. Stefani Show* podcast, and medical director of Wholehearted Integrative Psychiatry, Austin, TX

In *Live Beyond Your Label*, Erin offers hope and encouragement through sharing her own personal journey and lived experience with bipolar disorder, depression, and PTSD. Her LIVE framework for healing has a proven track record—she's been in remission herself for over a decade, and she's helped hundreds of clients do the same. Erin offers a gentle plan geared toward healing that's full of self-compassion. Her invitation feels familiar because *it is*: She reminds us of Jesus' invitation to an easy yoke and light burden—and the freedom that kind of life provides.

CAROLINE FAUSEL, NBC-HWC, creator of Olive You Whole and author of *A Simply Healthy Life*

Live Beyond Your Label is a must-read for anyone feeling trapped by the limitations of their diagnosis or self-imposed identity. This book beautifully bridges the gap between science and faith, offering practical tools to uncover the root issues of emotional and physical struggles. As a functional medicine physician, I deeply appreciate the holistic approach taken here—addressing stress, trauma, diet, movement, and mindset in a way that empowers and heals. If you're ready to break free from labels and step into the life you were meant to live, this book is your guide. Highly recommended!

DR. TABATHA BARBER, triple board-certified physician, author of *Fast to Faith*, and founder of the Fast to Faith Coaching Academy

LIVE BEYOND YOUR LABEL

A Holistic Approach to Breaking Old Patterns and
Rediscovering a Healthier You in Mind, Body, and Spirit

ERIN KERRY

TYNDALE
REFRESH
Think Well. Live Well. Be Well.

Visit Tyndale online at tyndale.com.

Visit Tyndale Refresh online at tyndalerefresh.com.

Tyndale, Tyndale's quill logo, *Tyndale Refresh*, and the Tyndale Refresh logo are registered trademarks of Tyndale House Ministries. Tyndale Refresh is a nonfiction imprint of Tyndale House Publishers, Carol Stream, Illinois.

Live Beyond Your Label: A Holistic Approach to Breaking Old Patterns and Rediscovering a Healthier You in Mind, Body, and Spirit

Copyright © 2025 by Erin Kerry. All rights reserved.

Cover photograph of abstract painting copyright © Donna Liu/Shutterstock. All rights reserved.

Author photograph copyright © 2023 by Katharine Elkins. All rights reserved.

Interior illustration of Colored Feeling Wheel by Feeling Wheel is licensed under a Creative Commons Attribution-Share-Alike 4.0 International License.

Cover design by Eva M. Winters

Interior design by Laura Cruise

Edited by Christine M. Anderson

Published in association with the literary agency of The Steve Laube Agency.

Unless otherwise indicated, all Scripture quotations are from The ESV® Bible (The Holy Bible, English Standard Version®), copyright © 2001 by Crossway, a publishing ministry of Good News Publishers. Used by permission. All rights reserved.

Scripture quotations marked CSB are taken from the Christian Standard Bible,® copyright © 2017 by Holman Bible Publishers. Used by permission. Christian Standard Bible® and CSB® are federally registered trademarks of Holman Bible Publishers.

Scripture quotations marked NIV are taken from the Holy Bible, *New International Version*,® *NIV*.® Copyright © 1973, 1978, 1984, 2011 by Biblica, Inc.® Used by permission. All rights reserved worldwide.

Scripture quotations marked NLT are taken from the *Holy Bible*, New Living Translation, copyright © 1996, 2004, 2015 by Tyndale House Foundation. Used by permission of Tyndale House Publishers, Carol Stream, Illinois 60188. All rights reserved.

Scripture quotations marked MSG are taken from *The Message*, copyright © 1993, 2002, 2018 by Eugene H. Peterson. Used by permission of NavPress. All rights reserved. Represented by Tyndale House Publishers.

The URLs in this book were verified prior to publication. The publisher is not responsible for content in the links, links that have expired, or websites that have changed ownership after that time.

For information about special discounts for bulk purchases, please contact Tyndale House Publishers at csresponse@tyndale.com, or call 1-855-277-9400.

Library of Congress Cataloging-in-Publication Data

A catalog record for this book is available from the Library of Congress.

ISBN 978-1-4964-9126-8

Printed in the United States of America

31	30	29	28	27	26	25
7	6	5	4	3	2	1

For Richard, my human GABA
(but not in a codependent way)

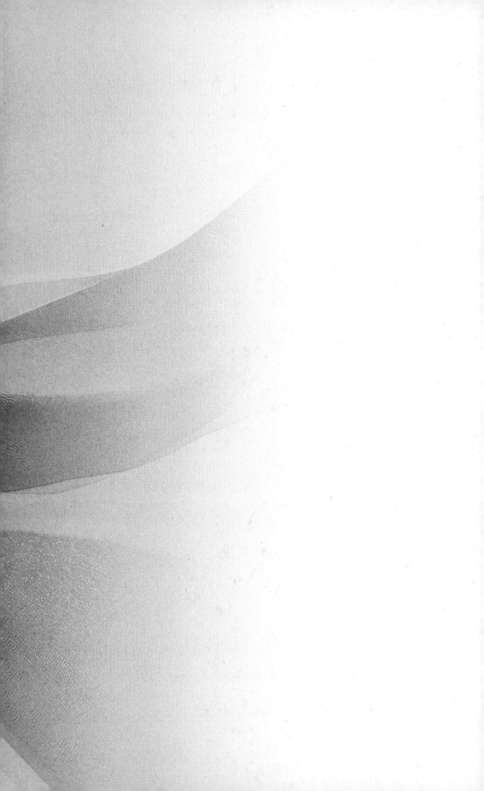

Disclaimer

The author has made every attempt to provide information that is accurate and complete, but this book is not intended as a substitute for professional medical advice. This book is not meant to be used, nor should it be used, to diagnose or treat any medical or psychological condition. Readers are advised to consult their own medical advisors whose responsibility it is to determine the condition of, and best treatment for, the reader.

The case examples in this book are composites based on the author's professional interactions with hundreds of clients over the years. All names are invented, and any resemblance between the composites and real people is coincidental.

Contents

       The Labels We Wear *1*
1. An Invitation to Examine the Label *9*

PART 1: **Learn to Address Stress** *23*
2. The Two Types of Stress Draining Us All *25*
3. How Your Self-Talk Impacts Your Health *39*
4. Could Your Pesky Thoughts Be Protective? *55*
5. Your Breath Reflects Your Stress Levels *69*

PART 2: **Identify the Root Issues** *81*
6. Is It Me or My Trauma Response? *83*
7. The Coping Mechanisms That Kept You Safe *99*
8. Unblocking Your Feelings *115*
9. Looking for a Magic Fix *127*

PART 3: **Add Variety to Your Diet** *139*
10. A Body in Stress Won't Digest *141*
11. Using Food to Support Your Mood *153*
12. Weight Issues and Restoring Body Peace *167*

PART 4: **Exercise Your Body and Brain** *181*
13. Engaging in Healthy Emotional Regulation *183*
14. Movement as Medicine *197*
15. Healing Through Rest *213*

       Labeled with Wholeness *227*
       Acknowledgments *230*
       Notes *235*
       About the Author *245*

The Labels We Wear

"You have manic-depressive illness, and you will struggle with this for the rest of your life."

Sitting in the psychiatrist's office with my parents, I was in complete denial as I listened to the latest explanation of my "broken brain." I'd already won the prize of PTSD. Depression and I had partied, too—and those meds made for a memorable party favor. Now, as an eighteen-year-old college freshman, I was being handed a new label: *bipolar*. I was officially unstable, the walking punchline of a joke about Texas weather. This label completely altered how I viewed myself for many years to follow.

My labels told me that my brain could not be trusted. Neither could my feelings. The next few years involved more meds. More attempts to sleep my sickness away. More struggle. I prayed to God to make me normal, and I frequently ranted my resentment about what he had allowed into my life. When he didn't come through for me in the ways I wanted, I took matters into my own hands, self-medicating with food, alcohol, and distractions. Filled with doubts about my identity, I picked up more labels. *Anxious. Hungry. Scattered. Overweight. Exhausted.*

When I became pregnant at twenty-two, yet another new label emerged—*single mom*. Unwed and unwanted. Alone. Knocked up, with a child out of wedlock.

It was a lot. A lot of labels. A lot of feelings. And *a lot* to process.

That was how my story began, but it's not how it continued. Slowly, over many years, I became empowered, learning to live beyond all the labels. Discovering how to listen to my body and advocate for myself set me on a journey to wholeness and healing—physically, emotionally, and spiritually.

An Invitation to Peace

If you've felt plagued by labels too, allow me to invite you on a journey toward peace. As a health coach who has been in remission from my illnesses for well over a decade, I hope to light a tiny spark in your heart, bringing you closer to wholeness and restoration. I work with women (and some men) of all ages and stages who wrestle with anxiety, depression, panic attacks, mood swings, fatigue, hormonal imbalances, trauma, autoimmune disease, metabolic dysfunction, disordered eating behaviors, body image issues, and so much more. Many of them feel stuck and discouraged by their lack of progress or their perceived inability to "get it together."

Statistics show that 26 percent of Americans will be diagnosed with a mental illness at some point in their lives.[1] Over 50 percent will be diagnosed with a chronic illness.[2] You may be one of the diagnosed, labeled for life—or it feels that way.

Or perhaps you've labeled yourself, using terms such as *overwhelmed, exhausted, too emotional, negative, needy, damaged, anxious,* or *addicted*. Maybe these labels have initially been helpful for you to make sense of your symptoms and life experiences. That's okay! Unfortunately, many labels can eventually become constraining, preventing you from living a life of integrated wholeness. The weight of these labels might have kept you from engaging in supportive relationships—whether with your heavenly Father, other people, or even yourself.

The invitation to "live beyond your label" doesn't mean pretending the labels are nonexistent or unimportant. In fact, addressing the labels may be a crucial part of determining how much of your identity has been formed by them. Identifying and examining your labels are necessary parts of the journey to wholeness. But living solely through the lens of labels can negatively impact how you live your life. Creating an identity based on labels leads to unhealthy compartmentalization of mind, body, and spirit—pitting parts of yourself against one another. And for many of us, being labeled can lead to overidentification with the corresponding symptoms. While a diagnosis doesn't equal a prognosis, labels can become negative self-fulfilling prophecies. Dr. Lissa Rankin writes, "By labeling a patient with a negative prognosis and robbing him or her of the hope that cure might be possible, we may ultimately prove the poor prognosis we have bestowed upon our patient correct."[3]

Living beyond your label means you can look at your label (and maybe even appreciate its function) without being defined by it. You can understand that while labels can give a name to a collection of presenting symptoms, they don't tell you how to manage the symptoms. When you live beyond your label, you can view your symptoms as interconnected pieces of a complex puzzle that makes you uniquely *you*. Assembling the puzzle pieces then becomes a catalyst that forges deeper connections within yourself and to the world around you. This helps you see that no matter your label—whether it's been given *to* you or *by* you—your life has a purpose, and so does your pain.

I struggled for years to make connections between my mental, emotional, spiritual, and physical health. I shoved away unpleasant symptoms so I could push through life, even if doing so numbed me too much in the process. But none of us can live a life of wholeness if we're living a life of compartmentalization. Made in the likeness of a three-in-one God (Father, Son, and Holy Spirit), you bear God's image in your body, mind, and spirit. Every part of you matters to God. No part of you is cut off from his transformational presence, no matter what label you've received. In fact, God uses your body, mind, and spirit to integrate wholeness into everything he's designed for you to be and do. Even the pesky symptoms you experience can alert you to a need for integrated wholeness.

I don't want you to simply address your symptoms. I want you to look beneath the symptoms, to dig into the roots of your labels and examine contributing factors—without judgment or criticism. This coaching method is what I use with my clients as well. It's an approach that comes from the field of functional medicine, and it completely altered the way I view my health, helping me to untangle decades of painful symptoms. The Institute for Functional Medicine defines this methodology as "a systems biology-based approach that focuses on identifying and addressing the root cause of disease. Each symptom or differential diagnosis may be one of many contributing to an individual's illness."[4]

Functional medicine allows us to look beyond our labels and peel back the contributing causes like the layers of an onion. For example, if a client is diagnosed with depression, I consider all the factors that might affect the manifestation of their diagnosis: lifestyle, genes, nutrition, sleep patterns, inflammation, medications, vitamin and/or mineral deficiencies, immune health, metabolism, digestive health, toxin exposure, hormones, or even surgeries. I imagine myself as something like a holistic detective, looking for patterns of imbalance so I can offer support through tools that bring healing to the mind, body, and spirit.

My Christian faith allows me to take an even more holistic view of functional medicine. God cares about your body, just as he cares about your mind and spirit. He created you with a body that he declared very good. He's given you one vessel to live out your purpose, and he's provided you with incredible tools within your body to seek homeostasis (balance). When the body is out of balance, it signals you with alerts. By honoring the design you've been given and partnering with it, you can better appreciate the Creator who put you together.

Through this method, I'll share what I discovered on my healing journey and how I have supported hundreds of clients with their own journeys. My favorite part about this is that it equips *you* to advocate for *you*.

Reading *Live Beyond Your Label*

Live Beyond Your Label is organized into four parts, according to the acronym LIVE, which represents the four foundational components of my coaching method:

Learn to address stress
Identify the root issues
Add *Variety* to your diet
Exercise your body and brain

Part 1, "Learn to Address Stress," explores the two types of stress everyone experiences and how they manifest in daily life. We'll focus on the mind-body connection and ways to support a healthy stress response in the body and brain by addressing thought patterns and incorporating new tools for calming, such as breath work.

Part 2, "Identify the Root Issues," focuses on how trauma, coping mechanisms, and blocked feelings may be at the root of your struggle to move forward in your healing journey. You'll learn how to view your journey with a fresh perspective, discovering tools to help you partner with and listen to your body, even when you feel like your body is working against you.

Part 3, "Add Variety to Your Diet," explores how stress hinders digestion of vital nutrients. You'll learn how to have a healthier relationship with food and your body as you continue to partner with it. We'll also consider a new perspective on the body weight conversation, and how even with weight fluctuations, your body is on your side, trying to protect you.

Part 4, "Exercise Your Body and Brain," focuses on practicing healthy emotional regulation to pursue peace with your own mental well-being and that of others. You'll learn how movement is an essential tool for shifting mood and see what kinds of movement practices can be therapeutic for different mood states. You'll discover how rest and sleep are not the same thing, but both are necessary for continued healing and growth.

The end of each chapter features activities to enable you to make the mind-body connection. These exercises are designed to help you connect what you've learned in a holistic way by showing you how to gently partner with your unique body and brain instead of fighting against them or forcing them to change.

I wrote *Live Beyond Your Label* because I want you to know that there is hope. The pages of this book brim with what I hope will be a fresh perspective and tools to support your healing journey. I share a lot of my own stories because I don't want you to feel alone in yours. My story also introduces tools I've used with hundreds of clients—people like you—whom I've coached and supported. You'll notice an emphasis on nutrition, movement, and rest, but in a far gentler way than you may be used to. My goal is to help you keep primary things primary—your relationship with God, your relationship with others, and your relationship with yourself.

As we travel together through this book, it's my prayer that you'll become increasingly empowered to look and live beyond your label. I hope you'll begin to view your life, and all your interconnected parts, with grace and self-compassion. I hope you'll stop beating yourself up, stop overthinking and self-judging. And I hope you'll give yourself permission to adopt a mindset of curiosity so you can learn to just *be*.

This book doesn't take the place of medical advice. It's not a substitute for medication, a wellness program, or your daily Bible reading. Consider it just another tool in your toolbox—one that will enable you to walk away empowered and advocating for yourself with a renewed perspective of your mind, body, and spirit.

Are you ready to start digging deep to unearth the roots of your labels? If so, I'm eager to be your companion on the journey. I, too, have been stuck in my stigma, overwhelmed by all the well-meaning health advice. I've been where you are, but I'm no longer there. I walk in the freedom that comes from living beyond my label.

You can too. Let's do this!

1

AN INVITATION TO EXAMINE THE LABEL

I lay sprawled across the center of my parents' king-size bed, waiting for the phone call from the doctor's office. The complete silence of the house, usually a comfort, made the waiting more ominous. The first pregnancy test was inconclusive. Too soon to tell. The exam at the doctor's office hadn't helped my anxiety. Echoes of the doctor's findings filled my head: "Your exam revealed internal abrasions and lacerations, indicative of rough intercourse or sexual assault. Do you want to file a report?"

File a report? How do I file a report about a night I don't remember? How do I explain months of self-destructive alcohol abuse combined with heavy psych meds that make memories unreliable? How do I explain to the doctor that I knew something bad was going to happen, and I was just waiting for the inevitable?

The ringing phone hijacked my downward spiral.

"Your results are in, and we want you to come to the office to hear our findings."

My mom came with me, and to my horror she had invited my dad to meet us at the office. I couldn't believe she'd asked him to be there. Maybe it comforted her, but it didn't soothe my cycling thoughts. *When Dad hears, it will confirm what he already knows about me: I'm a failure; I'm not the daughter he can be proud of. He'll be angry. He'll be embarrassed and ashamed of me. I failed him and everyone else. I'm the preacher's daughter who got knocked up.*

Sitting with my parents at the doctor's office, feeling completely alone, I listened in numb shock. *Pregnant.* My parents asked questions, and they heard the same exam report. Abrasions and lacerations. Hearing the words again, in the presence of my parents, brought me fear and shame.

And there was more. "Due to the nature of your psychiatric medication and the birth defects it causes, termination of the pregnancy may be advised."

No. I won't terminate the pregnancy. I didn't know what to do, but I knew that wasn't the option I wanted. It was the only thing I was clear about in that moment.

Back at my parents' house, before I'd gotten the call from the doctor's office, I'd received a different type of phone call. I'd answered it only because I thought it was the doctor's office.

"Erin, is that you?" asked my mom's friend Suzy, who sounded like she was in her car. "Can you look up a verse for me really fast?"

"Um, okay." Putting down the phone, I grabbed the nearest Bible, which wasn't far. My dad's sermon prep chair was to my right.

"Look up Zephaniah 3:17."

I opened to the passage and read it aloud: "The Lord your God is in your midst, a mighty one who will save; he will rejoice over you with gladness; he will quiet you by his love; he will exult over you with loud singing" (Zephaniah 3:17).

AN INVITATION TO EXAMINE THE LABEL

As I ended the phone call with Suzy, I felt a strange peace wash over my entire body. *Whatever happens, God is here. Whatever the results, he is with me.* The verse from Zephaniah became my anthem for the remainder of my pregnancy.

While many believed my mental instability was a red flag that precluded healthy parenting, I chose to keep and raise my baby girl, who was born healthy and whole. I gave her the name Isabel, which means "consecrated to God," because I wanted her to grow up knowing her life has meaning and purpose. And though she was a surprise to me, her life was no surprise to God. The pregnancy may have shocked my small-town church community, but it didn't shock God. He used her new life to bring *me* new life.

As a twenty-three-year-old single mom who was also managing mental health issues and working on a teaching certificate, I didn't fit into any category. The singles' group at church was filled with nonparents. The moms' group catered to stay-at-home moms with husbands. The small groups usually consisted of couples. My teacher coworkers were mostly single, living unencumbered by any responsibility beyond turning in lesson plans on time. My friends from college and high school were experiencing young adulthood the "normal" way—starting jobs, dating, and going out without first having to find childcare.

I was different. I wasn't normal. *I was alone.*

The label *alone* framed most of my story and core belief system up to that point. I had given myself that label long ago—before the unexpected pregnancy, before the label *bipolar* was handed to me at eighteen, and before *depressed* was plastered on me in eighth grade. I carried that label even before the event I experienced at age nine that garnered me yet another label: *traumatized* with *PTSD*.

Alone weighed down my feet like cinder blocks, stemming from trauma and a belief that nobody really understood my feelings or my fear. Add to that the three scary-sounding diagnostic labels—*PTSD*, *depression*, and *bipolar* disorder—and it's not hard to see how my identity was overburdened with labels by the time I was eighteen.

What Are Labels and How Do We Get Them?

Labels are the shorthand ways we identify ourselves in a world that is constantly changing. They can be positive or negative and may be based on any number of things, such as personality traits, appearance, behaviors, health, social status, or experiences. Positive labels that affirm our strengths, skills, and relational connections can help us understand our role in the world and help us make meaning from difficult circumstances. Labels can explain personality traits and why we do the things we do. For example, I'm very extroverted, so it's hard for me to decline invitations to social events, but I also burn out easily. Labels also help us make sense of our actions and even how we relate to one another. For example, one of my labels is *firstborn*, a neutral label that is simply a fact but also one that reveals something about my identity. Like many firstborns, I see the need for efficiency and problem-solving. I tend to overperform and have a strong sense of personal responsibility to make sure others are "okay." Knowing that these are common traits for firstborns helps me understand the *why* behind how I show up for others.

Unfortunately, many of the labels we give ourselves are negative rather than positive. Negative labels limit and undermine our strengths, skills, and relational connections. They keep us stuck— in hopelessness, self-defeating behaviors, or toxic relationships. Negative labels can also become core beliefs or identity statements that hold us back from living out our God-given purpose.

Whether we pick them up in childhood, adolescence, or adulthood, we all have labels. Some of them we give ourselves, and some

What Are Core Beliefs?

Core beliefs are deeply rooted beliefs we all have, usually emerging from childhood, that impact how we see ourselves, the world, and the role we play in it. Just as labels can be positive, neutral, or negative, so can core beliefs. One of the things that makes beliefs "core" is their rigidity, sometimes even in the face of evidence to the contrary. For example, we might believe we are unlovable even when others consistently demonstrate their love for us. Or we might believe our worth depends on our performance or achievement and feel we are worth more when we succeed and less when we fail.

Core beliefs don't exist as thoughts alone; they also exist in the biochemistry of the brain. In fact, core beliefs can become so entrenched in the neural networks of the brain that we interpret every life experience as confirming our core beliefs even when that may not be the case. That's why it can be very difficult for us to accept or even consider any information that contradicts our core beliefs. Core beliefs become part of our internal operating system, influencing everything from self-perception and behaviors to decision-making and relationships.

are given to us by others. Three of the most common kinds of labels are diagnostic labels, experiential labels, and self-assigned labels.

Diagnostic Labels

Diagnostic labels are given by medical or mental health care practitioners. The purpose of giving a condition a diagnostic label is to identify the most effective treatment plan for relief of symptoms and for healing. Some of my clients experience relief when they get a diagnosis. For example, when Amy's doctor diagnosed her with obsessive-compulsive disorder (OCD), she felt validated. It gave her a framework to understand her condition and propelled her to seek support. Our coaching sessions helped her create habits to minimize the stress that overwhelmed her self-protective, hypervigilant brain.[1]

Unfortunately, diagnostic labels can sometimes create unintentional confusion. This can happen when medical or mental health conditions are misdiagnosed or when there doesn't appear to be any clear diagnosis. Diagnoses can be especially difficult for mental health disorders because they are based on a cluster of symptoms over a specific period. There is no blood test for trauma; there is no brain scan or lab work to determine if someone has depression or bipolar disorder. The diagnoses are based on symptoms alone—and symptoms can often mimic other disorders.[2]

Consider my client Kelly, who struggled with her diagnosis. Having grown up experiencing repeated trauma, she went on to marry a man who was verbally and emotionally abusive. When her mental health symptoms became too much for her, she sought the help of four psychiatrists over a period of years and received a different diagnosis from each one. One said her problems were psychosomatic—all in her head. Another told her she met the criteria for bipolar disorder. Another told her it was her thyroid creating the symptoms. And yet another diagnosed her with both bipolar disorder and ADHD. *What in the world?* All Kelly wanted was respite from her symptoms. What she received was more confusion and a whole bunch of labels that provided no relief from her struggles.

Identifying and living with a diagnostic label can be challenging, often requiring nuanced conversations with medical and mental health care professionals. I struggled to understand myself for many years after being diagnosed with PTSD, depression, and bipolar disorder. What aspects of my behavior were symptoms of an illness, and what was just me being me? Here's what I've found to be true for me and for those I work with: If getting a diagnosis brings you the support and tools you need, awesome! If not, then maybe it's time to get curious about new ways to advocate for your mental and physical health so your diagnosis doesn't keep you from living a full life.

AN INVITATION TO EXAMINE THE LABEL

Experiential Labels

All your experiences—positive and negative—shape your identity. However, trauma not only shapes your identity, but it also redefines the world and alters your perception of it, sometimes permanently. As physician and trauma expert Gabor Maté states, "Whether we realize it or not, it is our woundedness, or how we cope with it, that dictates much of our behavior, shapes our social habits, and informs our ways of thinking about the world."[3]

One of the ways trauma can permanently alter our perception of the world is by tricking us into believing it's not safe to feel safe—even when it is safe. My client Jamie experienced this as a result of growing up in a home where there wasn't enough food. She was the youngest in her large family, and finances were tight. By the time the big kids grabbed food, she was left with little and often went to bed hungry. As an adult, she struggled with overeating. She couldn't get enough because there was always the what-if question in the back of her mind. *What if I don't get more tomorrow? What if I won't ever have this specific type of food again?* Her childhood trauma labeled her *hungry*, *impulsive*, and *unfulfilled*. As a result, she felt addicted to food.

Even the negative experiences you may view as "not that bad" can leave a lasting imprint on your nervous system, altering the lens through which you view the world. Maybe you were bullied in middle school and some of those taunts remain with you today, creating a label such as *loser*, *reject*, or *outcast*. Maybe you experienced sexual harassment, but others brushed it aside or even laughed it off, so you blamed yourself, creating a label from that scenario—*tease*, *flirt*, or even worse, *whore*. Maybe you always felt somewhat anxious but didn't want to burden anyone, so you stuffed it down, creating a label—*nervous wreck*, *high-strung*, or *scattered*.

Whether or not you've experienced what you would consider trauma, you've no doubt experienced some form of adversity in your life. And those experiences shape how you perceive yourself and the world around you. Those adverse experiences likely caused you to create new labels.

Self-Assigned Labels

Most of us say some pretty mean things to ourselves. In fact, the habit of negative self-talk is often so deeply entrenched in who we are and how we go through life that we barely realize we're doing it anymore. Self-talk creates our labels. These labels inform our narratives and become themes in our stories that can shape our behaviors and decisions in self-defeating ways.

You may think your self-given labels are all in your head, but the truth is they're also in your body. Your thoughts are chemical messages that get broadcast through your bodily systems. "Thoughts are real things," writes Dr. Caroline Leaf, a neuroscience researcher. "And, like all real things, they generate energy: little packets of energy called photons, which are the fundamental particles of light."[4] The labels you give yourself, whether based on your diagnoses, experiences, or self-talk, can impact your physical health, even leading to accelerated aging. Dr. Leaf points out, "If we don't manage our minds, the organs in our physical bodies will get older than our actual chronological age."[5] When you give yourself a negative label and live tethered to that label, it is detrimental to your mental *and* physical health. Creating an entire identity based on a label may even limit your ability to live the abundant life that God has planned for you.

This is not to say that you are somehow to blame for your mental or physical health concerns. You are not. But there is an undisputed connection between your mind and your body. And just as your body tries to protect you with symptoms that sometimes become problematic, your patterns of thinking do the same.

AN INVITATION TO EXAMINE THE LABEL

My client Patricia labeled herself *lazy* and *unmotivated* when, as a young child, she struggled to keep up with schoolwork and zoned out during lessons. Her parents knew she was struggling, but this happened long before quiet, well-mannered girls were given diagnoses of ADHD. Patricia believed if she tried harder, she'd get better. After failing throughout her educational years, she resigned herself to the fact that school wasn't for her. Calling herself lazy and unmotivated was her way of protecting herself from more failure. By the time she made an appointment with me to get help managing stress hormones, she was in her fifties but still beating herself up for her lack of dedication as a child, which only amplified her stress.

Like Patricia, you may have given yourself labels to understand yourself better or to make sense of your behaviors. That's very common! Unfortunately, it becomes problematic when the label you've made for yourself becomes your identity and holds you back from living in the truth of who God says you are.

Understanding your labels and where they come from is essential for your healing journey. When you can identify the labels that weigh you down, you can prevent them from becoming a false identity.

You Are Not Your Label

I hear identity statements like these from my clients all the time:

> "I know it's just my anxiety talking, but . . ."
> "Sorry about the rabbit trail. Ignore my ADHD brain—I'm back on track now."
> "My mom's bipolar, and I'm bipolar. I'll never have it together."

What Labels Have You Been Given?

Place a check mark next to any words that describe a label that was given to you—by yourself or someone else.

- ☐ ADHD
- ☐ depressed
- ☐ anxious
- ☐ negative
- ☐ bipolar
- ☐ heavy
- ☐ obsessive-compulsive
- ☐ weird
- ☐ sick
- ☐ imposter
- ☐ failure
- ☐ overachiever
- ☐ perfectionist
- ☐ emotional
- ☐ unstable
- ☐ stressed
- ☐ dramatic
- ☐ triggered
- ☐ broken
- ☐ hungry
- ☐ boring
- ☐ addicted
- ☐ impulsive
- ☐ unworthy
- ☐ unlovable
- ☐ not enough
- ☐ different
- ☐ loser
- ☐ weak
- ☐ helpless
- ☐ exhausting
- ☐ tired
- ☐ invisible
- ☐ alone
- ☐ traumatized
- ☐ needy
- ☐ other: _____

The last example is particularly difficult for me to hear. As someone who's been diagnosed with bipolar disorder and suffered for many years before finding stability, I understand how easy it is for a diagnosis to become an identity. For some reason, people seem to feel free to make identity-defining jokes about bipolar disorder especially. "Oh, did you hear? She's bipolar, so that explains it." It's hard to imagine someone saying, "You're acting depression" or, "You're acting anxiety" in the same way they say, "You're acting bipolar."

Bipolar disorder is an illness someone has, not an adjective. Like other mental illnesses, it is diagnosed from a set of symptoms presenting for a period of time. Contrary to what is often represented, most bipolar sufferers have only one to two mood cycles per year. It's not a permanent state of being, or even a semipermanent state of mood swings. Yet it is deeply misunderstood, leading others to make identity statements that are both inaccurate and

AN INVITATION TO EXAMINE THE LABEL

harmful. Please hear my heart: If you have been diagnosed with bipolar disorder or any other mental health condition, you have a medical diagnosis of a disorder and you exhibit symptoms of an illness—but you are *not* your illness.

Equating our identity with our struggles is such a human thing to do. It's how we seek to make meaning of our messes and confusion. *Why did this happen to me? Because I am my label. Why do I have these problems? Because I am my label. Why don't I fit in? Because I am my label.* It's a pretty efficient system for making sense of things, right? And yet it's also a lie.

No matter what you've been told or what you've told yourself, you are not your label. Your label is not your identity—and you don't have to be limited by it. What you struggle with may impact how you function, but your label doesn't define you or diminish your value and worth. If you find that hard to believe or accept right now, that's okay. Especially after years of struggle, it can be difficult to separate your identity from your symptoms. But it is vitally important to do so. And I can promise you that it *is* possible—not just because I've experienced it personally and helped others to do the same, but because this freedom is rooted in a foundational truth of Scripture.

Thanks to Jesus, you are not your label. Because of the grace and belonging you have in him, you have a new identity—a lasting identity that never changes, despite the diagnosis, the trauma, and what you tell yourself. Your foundational identity is this: *You are a child of God* (see 1 John 3:2). This identity is unchanging—no matter your diagnostic, experiential, and self-assigned labels.

If your story is like mine or that of some of my clients, your labels have probably built up over a lifetime. You likely carry heavy wounds, sorrow, shame, and more. Perhaps the thought of even acknowledging your labels feels overwhelming. If so, I invite you to receive these words as the Lord's invitation just for you:

> Are you tired? Worn out? Burned out on religion? Come to me. Get away with me and you'll recover your life. I'll show you how to take a real rest. Walk with me and work with me—watch how I do it. Learn the unforced rhythms of grace. I won't lay anything heavy or ill-fitting on you. Keep company with me and you'll learn to live freely and lightly.
> MATTHEW 11:28-30, MSG

Jesus doesn't burden you with anything that doesn't fit and isn't supposed to be there. Instead of labels, Jesus offers you identity markers such as *loved, redeemed, precious, forgiven, gifted, empowered,* and *freed*. As a new creation in him, as a child in his Kingdom, you already have a premium identity. When you identify first with who you are in Christ, you no longer have to carry the burden of identifying with your label or its limitations.

Learning to live into your new identity in Christ isn't a linear process; no healing process is. And I'm not going to sugarcoat it: Learning to live beyond your label is hard work. There are no shortcuts. It takes courage to break with old patterns, address stress, and identify your triggers. Implementing change with new tools requires determination. But there *is* relief that comes from awareness and change. And if you're willing to work through your discomfort and dig deeper into the root of your struggles, you *can* experience freedom from the burden of your label.

MAKING THE MIND-BODY CONNECTION

To help you start recognizing the ways in which your mind influences your body, and your body influences your mind, I invite you to try the following exercise. To begin, use the prompts on the next page to learn how to pay attention to your body. Then listen to your body as you identify and examine your labels.

AN INVITATION TO EXAMINE THE LABEL

- *Pay attention to your body.* Your body is always sending you signals in response to your thoughts, but you might not always notice. You can practice paying attention to your body any time by noticing felt sensations in four areas: the head, stomach, chest, and back. If reading those four body parts makes you think of the children's song "Head, Shoulders, Knees, and Toes," and if using that melody helps you remember "Head, stomach, chest, and back"—go for it!

  › *Head.* You might notice tension in your head, jaw, neck, or face. Perhaps you have been clenching your teeth a lot, creating tension throughout your jaw.

  › *Stomach.* You may feel butterflies in the pit of your stomach or like you're about to plummet from the peak of a roller coaster. Maybe you have some cramping or tightness in your abdomen.

  › *Chest.* You might be aware of tightness in your chest, feel like it's difficult to take a deep breath, or notice your heart pounding.

  › *Back.* You may feel discomfort in your back, anywhere from the upper to lower portion or any of the sides. Perhaps you feel some pinching sensations or soreness from overexertion.

  As you pay attention to each felt sensation, try to describe it more specifically. For example, does it feel like light flutters or strong pricks? Is it buzzy or wavy? Is it fleeting or long-lasting? Is it soft or heavy, hot or cold, tight or loose, close or far away? What other ways can you describe the sensation?

Try to maintain awareness of your body as you work through the next part of this exercise, which is to identify your labels. Noticing felt sensations that certain words bring up for you is a useful tool to help you partner with your body and pay attention to its signals.

- **Identify your labels**. Consider which label(s) you identify with, including diagnostic labels, experiential labels, and self-assigned labels.

  › *Make a list*. Use a journal or a pad of paper to write down as many labels as come to mind. If you're uncertain what your labels might be, begin by reviewing the list in "What Labels Have You Been Given?" (page 18).

  › *Narrow down your list*. Briefly review your list and circle the one or two labels you struggle with most.

  › *Examine your label(s)*. Consider each of the labels you circled from the perspective of an interested observer. Pick them up one at a time, like you're picking up an interesting rock on a nature trail. Turn them over and notice what you notice without judgment or harsh words. Allow yourself to be curious about what you see. For example:

  > *My label of not enough plays a pretty big role in my life. I wonder how much that's impacting me?*

  > *My label of dramatic causes me to feel pretty negative toward myself.*

  > *I have more labels than I thought I did. I wonder how they show up in my daily interactions?*

  > *I notice that I have both diagnostic labels and self-assigned labels. I feel more bothered by the labels I give myself than the diagnostic ones. That's interesting.*

- **Notice your body.** What felt sensations, if any, were you aware of as you worked through your labels? Or what felt sensations are you aware of now? The goal is to simply notice what you notice.

PART 1

LEARN TO ADDRESS STRESS

IDENTIFY the root issues

add VARIETY to your diet

EXERCISE your body and brain

When I sit down with new clients, I ask a lot of questions about their lives. Even though they've already filled out several intake forms detailing their full health history, I review their information with them verbally, wanting to hear how they describe patterns and practices in their own words. While every individual's struggle is unique, when it comes down to it, there's an overarching theme of stress for everyone I talk to.

As humans, we all share a need for safety and connection. Persistent, unmanaged stress is often the catalyst that ruptures our sense of safety and ability to connect wholeheartedly to God, others, and ourselves. Stress that isn't managed creates an emotional and physiological disconnect that keeps us stuck and frustrated with ourselves.

In part 1, we'll explore the full picture of *why* stress drives dysfunction and *how* looking at your stressors helps you take the necessary steps to manage them. Your body constantly sends you "dashboard alerts" through symptoms, whether you ignore them and hit the gas pedal harder or choose to pull over for a checkup. My hope is that when you see how beautifully interconnected all parts of your body and its systems are, you'll feel empowered to tune in to your unique needs and learn to address stress.

2

THE TWO TYPES OF STRESS DRAINING US ALL

I wasn't supposed to be depressed. I shouldn't have been sad.

From the outside looking in, everything in my thirteen-year-old life appeared fine. But on the inside, I was dying. Late at night in my bedroom, I filled pages and pages of my journal with feelings of darkness. The gloom of depression suffocated me like a heavy winter coat in the middle of a Texas summer. It clouded my perception, especially when I was by myself. I was trying to keep it together with activities and friendships and typical teenage drama. But I didn't want to be alive. In fact, I wanted to go to sleep and not wake up for a long, long time. Maybe ever.

Externally, I wore a mask of happiness. Internally, I felt broken, empty, and alone in my suffering. The disconnect between my outer life and my inner darkness made the depression much worse. I wanted to snap out of it but couldn't, and I felt guilty for being depressed. The shame of feeling sad was a burden. I tried praying it away, but the sadness persisted. There was something wrong with me, something broken deep inside. The harder I tried to keep up the facade of happiness, the more depleted I felt.

Looking back, I grieve for that young girl. The journey to healing that followed was long and difficult. I spent many years seeking relief from the mental instability that plagued me. When sadness crept in, anxiety and racing thoughts picked up speed and the highs of hypomania could hit me at any moment. Even when I did the "right things," such as taking meds, exercising, and trying to eat healthy, I still felt scattered and exhausted. I longed for a magic fix—a cure that would give me a sense of stability and help me to feel normal again. Instead, I felt chronically depleted both mentally and physically.

What I didn't know at the time was that my symptoms told a story—that they were screaming about the state of my internal and external environments, trying to tell me that I was in a state of severe stress.

Redefining Stress

Stress is ubiquitous in contemporary life,[1] and the word gets tossed around as if we all understand what it means. Most of us routinely talk about the daily kinds of stress we experience—in our work, finances, parenting, commuting, and social concerns. Then there is the stress we experience from larger issues, such as life changes, unexpected challenges, or tragic events. In all these situations, we tend to think of stress primarily as an emotional experience—specifically, the worry or tension we feel in a difficult scenario. But stress isn't just emotional; it's also physiological.

According to the Cleveland Clinic, "Stress is the natural reaction your body has when changes or challenges occur. It can result in many different physical, emotional and behavioral responses."[2] Stress is not always a bad thing. In fact, acute or short-term stressors can create resilience. One example is *eustress*, which is a moderate stress we experience from positive changes or from learning a new skill; we feel brief discomfort from the challenge, but the overall experience is enjoyable and motivates us to keep going. *Hormetic stress* is another type of stress that is challenging to the body but not depleting. Working out is an example of a hormetic stressor. We experience a brief period of physical stress to increase strength and cardiovascular health, which reaps a plethora of benefits—then we recover afterward.

When you experience emotional stress, your brain alerts your body that there's a threat. Your body doesn't know the difference between a real or perceived threat—whether the threat is a charging bear or an upcoming work presentation—so it picks up on the signals of unsafety and responds accordingly. Maybe your heart rate speeds up, your blood pressure spikes, or your digestion slows. During an acutely stressful situation, you might start to sweat or experience shallow, rapid breathing.

As unpleasant as these physiological responses might be, they are a *good* thing—evidence that your body is responding to your brain's cues and taking action to protect you. A threat triggers a release of adrenaline that increases your heart rate, delivering more blood flow to your brain and muscles, which makes you more alert. It also raises blood sugar levels to give you more energy. It's your body's way of preparing to respond to whatever the threat may be, enabling you to fight it or flee it. Your body's stress response is part of a physiological network of communication you need for survival. God designed your body this way to help you pay attention to and care for this vessel you've been given to live out your purpose. That's the good news about your stress response—it's protective.

However, your stress response also takes a toll on your body. That same release of adrenaline that enables you to escape a threat can also lead to hormonal imbalances and digestive distress. And when short-term stress becomes prolonged stress, it can lead to nutrient depletions. Just two hours of emotional stress can alter the composition of your gut microbiome, which impacts how your body synthesizes neurotransmitters (the chemical messengers that affect how you feel).[3] One week of constant emotional stress can deplete essential vitamins and minerals by up to 40 percent.[4] Your body stores only two days' worth of amino acids from protein. Because amino acids are crucial for creating neurotransmitters—including those that are calming, such as GABA—depleting them through prolonged stress can make it physiologically impossible for you to calm yourself or regulate your emotional response. There is no bottomless buffet of nutrients in your body—especially when you're stressed.

Perhaps you're beginning to see why learning to address stress is such a crucial component of getting to the root of your physical and mental health battles. Knowing what your stressors are and how they affect your physical and emotional well-being is essential for your healing journey. You can't remove all the stressors in your life, but you absolutely can learn to manage them differently. You can play offense instead of defense.

Two Types of Stress

Throughout my own health journey and in working with my clients, I've noticed there are consistently two types of stress draining us all: emotional stress and physiological stress. The stress may begin as acute, but it can quickly become chronic. Both types of stress create imbalances in the body, but they are triggered by different sources—one by the mind and the other by the body. Understanding both types can help us learn to better manage stress—before it manages us.

Is Stress Depleting You?

Place a check mark next to any of the following statements that resonate with you.

- ☐ I feel low on energy, hangry, or moody, or I experience brain fog if I don't eat regularly.
- ☐ Even when I get eight hours of sleep, I don't feel rested.
- ☐ I occasionally experience body soreness and tension in my shoulders and neck.
- ☐ I've lost interest in things that used to bring joy.
- ☐ Extreme temperature changes tend to throw off my mood.
- ☐ I struggle to transition from one thing to the next without feeling like I'm forgetting something in between.
- ☐ It's hard for me to relax or loosen up.
- ☐ I crave carbs, sugar, or alcohol to relax and calm down.
- ☐ I experience menstrual irregularities.
- ☐ I sometimes have feelings of hopelessness or loneliness.
- ☐ I often experience an urge to lie down and rest in the afternoon.
- ☐ I tend to shake when I feel nervous or under pressure.
- ☐ I force myself to keep going, but I feel like I'm always in survival mode.

Every statement you checked could be an alert your body is giving you, indicating through symptoms that stress is creating depletions in your body.

Emotional Stress Is Brain-Based Stress

Emotional stress is the type of stress we're most familiar with. We experience emotional stress when an external trigger impacts our emotional well-being. Another way to look at emotional stress is to think of it as brain-based stress. We feel it mentally first, and because that's overwhelming enough, we rarely recognize or acknowledge the impact it has on us physically.

Emotional stress may be caused by any number of things: toxic relationships, a negative work environment, burnout, trauma, grief, parenting challenges, technology overexposure, spiritual disconnect, a health diagnosis, a negative self-concept, or negative beliefs about the world. Being in a toxic relationship is *stressful*. Working for a narcissistic boss is *stressful*. Being diagnosed with a health condition is *stressful*. All of these are stressors we can recognize and understand.

I experienced many emotional stressors that led to my early life journey with depression. As a toddler, I experienced medical trauma when my lungs collapsed 75 percent, which caused me to question my safety in the world. My childhood was marked by asthma attacks, which left me feeling even less safe. At age nine, I witnessed the death of my grandfather on my front lawn due to anaphylaxis, an allergic reaction from shellfish cross contamination. His sudden death solidified my belief that the world was unpredictable and unsafe, and I was alone in it. So when my PTSD symptoms began to look like depression in eighth grade, it was a natural response to years of brewing despair and hopelessness due to emotional stressors.

Such unrelenting emotional stress brings unsafety to the body. Remember when I said the body doesn't know the difference between a real or perceived threat? When emotional stress is ongoing, the body intentionally creates ongoing imbalances as a form of protection. The body always prioritizes survival. If your body gets chronic signals of hypervigilance from your brain, your body will develop a corresponding hypervigilant response. This may include conserving fuel by lowering your metabolic rate, spiking blood pressure, amping up anxiety to give you a "wired but tired" feeling, or other changes. These alterations can cause unpleasant symptoms, so you might head to the doctor's office, not realizing that these symptoms are your body's dashboard alerts to that unending road trip of emotional stress.

Physiological Stress Is Body-Based Stress

Physiological stress occurs when there is an imbalance within the body's systems. While emotional stress is brain-based, physiological stress is body-based. It's a stress we first experience physically rather than mentally. When the body meets physiological stress, it doesn't feel safe to function optimally, so it creates unpleasant alerts, such as enhanced intestinal permeability (also known as "leaky gut"), blood sugar dysregulation, and ongoing digestive discomfort. Those alerts can eventually become mental health conditions that turn into labels, such as depression, anxiety, or bipolar disorder. Or they can develop into chronic disease diagnoses, such as autoimmune diseases, type 2 diabetes, or irritable bowel syndrome (IBS).

Examples of physiological stressors include some that might surprise you, such as ultra-processed foods and refined sugar, caffeine and energy drinks, nutrient deficiencies, and commonly prescribed medications. They also include microbial overgrowths or imbalances in the gut, exposure to toxins or allergens, lack of movement or too much high-intensity exercise, chronic low-calorie diets, and lack of sleep.

Anything that wreaks havoc on the physical body or impairs its functioning can make the body feel unsafe. It will impact energy availability, cognitive function, and even emotional health. And physiological stress most definitely impacts how we show up for our God-given purpose in the world.

My childhood was packed with physiological stressors, including mold exposure, chronic antibiotic use, chronic viruses and bacterial infections such as strep throat, asthma medications that were lifesaving but depleted nutrients, and intense sugar cravings and food obsession. I rarely felt well for long. As an overachieving firstborn who thrived on challenge, I stayed busy intellectually—always reading and questioning—to make up for the physical depletions I experienced. But I was tapped out at every level. Due to an irregular menstrual cycle, I was prescribed birth control pills, which we now know increase the risk of depression in teens by 130 percent.[5] When my depression surfaced in eighth grade, it was my body's way of telling me it was completely worn down.

Because physiological stress is experienced first in the body, we don't always recognize it or even know it's happening. Are we tired because our work schedule is demanding, or are we tired because we skip meals to keep working, limiting the availability of nutrients that give us energy? Are we having panic attacks due to relationship issues, or are we experiencing symptoms of blood sugar dysregulation?

One way to understand the impact of physiological stressors is to examine the impact of nutrient deficiencies. Because we live in an incredible time in history when food is readily available to most (especially in the US), we don't think we have deficiencies. Ironically, we even have medications to help people feel *less* hungry (imagine trying to explain this to your Depression-era great-grandparents). However, it may surprise you to learn that some of the food you're consuming may *not* be providing your body with nutrients that create energy. That's because at least 60 percent of the average American diet is comprised of ultra-processed foods.[6] These are foods that contain ingredients manufactured from whole foods, but they've been processed with additives, preservatives, and artificial colors and flavors, and reassembled to create shelf-stable, convenient meals. Ultra-processed foods by nature lack nutrients, contain ingredients that are stressful to digest, and are designed to hook us through "hyperpalatability"—that's the addictive "betcha can't have just one" quality.[7] The consequence is that many of us are undernourished. One study found that "94.3 percent of the US population do not meet the daily requirement for vitamin D, 88.5 percent for vitamin E, 52.2 percent for magnesium,

44.1 percent for calcium, 43.0 percent for vitamin A, and 38.9 percent for vitamin C."[8]

These ultra-processed foods contain refined carbohydrates and sugar that also create a rapid cycle of hungry-fed-hungry that sends the body on a physiological joyride I call the blood sugar roller coaster. The rapid rise and fall of blood sugar levels creates a stress response, releasing adrenaline (a fast-acting hormone needed for emergencies) as well as cortisol (a slow-acting hormone that regulates your body's response to long-term stress). When blood sugar rises and falls dramatically, it sends out more stress signals that impact your emotional and physical health. Sadly, it's a vicious cycle. As one researcher states, "Eating too many of the wrong carbohydrates too often causes a rise in stress hormones that urge us to eat to stabilize our metabolism."[9]

That's physiological stress.

The Compound Effect of Both Types of Stress

The dynamic duo of emotional and physiological stress often feed off one another, compounding the overall load. Although we are equipped to handle some level of routine stress, each of us has a different sized stress capacity bucket. When stressors fill up our bucket too fast, it reaches a tipping point. This is known as the allostatic load of stress.[10] It's what happens when the cumulative burdens of chronic stress exceed our ability to cope, resulting in chronic illness.

Take my client Julia, for example. Like me, she battled depression as a teenager and young adult. But she married a man who was controlling and routinely denigrated her with piercing statements that caused her to always feel "less than." The IBS symptoms she'd struggled with since childhood worsened until she got to the point where she experienced uncomfortable bloating with every meal. When we ran a food sensitivity test, the results indicated her body had developed adverse reactions to just about every one of her frequently consumed foods!

Did Julia's IBS symptoms (physiological stress) trigger her depression, or did her depression and marriage (emotional stress) trigger her worsening IBS symptoms and subsequent food reactions? This is an all-too-common question in my office for an all-too-common scenario. What came first? And how do we resolve it?

You and I were created with a holistic design—an integration of body and mind. It goes against our very design to separate the impact of the mind on the body and the body on the mind. Addressing these types of stressors and restoring balance require taking a holistic approach. And it starts with my favorite concept: nourishment.

Primary and Secondary Nourishment: The Antidote to Stress

I love the word *nourishment* and speak of it often when I give talks, teach classes, and coach clients. At its most fundamental definition, nourishment is "the food or other substances necessary for growth, health, and good condition."[11] When most of us consider nourishment, we tend to think of food. But look at that definition again. It mentions food or "other substances." Our *primary* nourishment doesn't come from the food we eat. Our primary nourishment comes from our most foundational relationships.[12]

Primary nourishment is the sustenance we receive when we feel securely attached to God, others, and ourselves. Primary nourishment restores safety to the body and brain by providing positive answers to questions such as, *Do you feel safe and connected in the world? Do you have what you need to respond to threats? Do you feel that your relationship needs are met?* When you feel safe in your relationships—when you know you are fully seen and fully loved—your brain is better able to filter out threats. When you know your purpose, feel supported, and understand your role in a larger story, your stress response changes.

Secondary nourishment is the sustenance we receive from nourishing food, enjoyable activities, hydration, sunshine, rest, and movement. Secondary nourishment brings physiological safety to the body, and it helps to counter the effects of both emotional and physiological stress. Meeting such basic human needs is essential for better emotional regulation. I don't know about you, but I get an extra dose of brain fog if I don't sleep well. When I'm not engaging my body in regular movement, my anxiety increases because I don't have an outlet for it. And don't even talk to me if I haven't had some uninterrupted alone time on the weekend to read in my cozy bed. Those are all ways I receive secondary nourishment.

Primary nourishment and secondary nourishment are both antidotes to the chronic stress problem. And just as emotional and physiological stress impact each other, primary and secondary nourishment are affected by each other.

I often say that a body in stress won't digest. When you're living in a chronic stress response, constantly reacting to emotional and physiological stressors, even the way you receive nutrition changes. That's why I consider food to be secondary nutrition. Yes, food can contribute to a healing environment, but your mindset while eating impacts how your body utilizes those nutrients.

The body won't feel safe to heal if it's not in a well-nourished environment—an environment in which you are fueled by your relationship with God first, but also by healthy relationships with others and yourself. Patterns of overscheduling, constant activities, negative self-talk, pushing through, ignoring symptoms, suppressing emotions, and neglecting spiritual practices will never foster the nourishment your soul truly craves.

Just as deficiencies in primary nourishment can impair the body's ability to receive secondary nourishment, the reverse is also true. When secondary nourishment needs aren't being met and there are imbalances (such as a poor sleep schedule, lack of movement, or lack of nutrients), the body won't get the signals it needs to support healthy emotional balance and positive relationships.

Remember my client, Julia, who developed IBS? Because she was depleted by emotional and physiological stress, she needed both primary and secondary nourishment to heal. Fortunately, she saw a therapist who helped her receive primary nourishment by addressing her thought life and her abusive marriage. In her sessions with me, we worked on secondary nourishment by removing the top foods triggering distress and implementing mindful eating practices, supplements, and nutritious foods to restore health to her digestive system. As her body began to benefit from secondary nourishment, her improved health helped her to better manage her emotional stress. And as her life got better, she began to feel truly seen by the one who provides true, lasting nourishment.

Your heavenly Father is the water of life and the nourisher of your soul. He longs to meet you in your stress desert and bring you to life. It may take some time, just as it did for Julia and as it did for me, but I can promise that he longs to restore, refresh, and renew you from the inside out—no matter where you find yourself today. He can be trusted to meet you in your wilderness of overwhelm.

MAKING THE MIND-BODY CONNECTION

- *Do a body scan to check for stress.* Take five to ten minutes to be completely still in a comfortable place where you won't be distracted.

  › Close your eyes, inhale deeply through your nose, and slowly exhale from your mouth, until your lungs are completely empty of air. As you breathe in, imagine filling a balloon with everything stressing you out right now. As you breathe out, picture that balloon deflating. Do this at least three to five times.

› Check in with yourself by taking notice of any parts of your body that feel different than others in some way. Notice especially your head, stomach, chest, and back. Are you experiencing "alerts" of stress in these areas?

› What parts of you are holding tightness or tension? Visualize breathing into those areas specifically as you take a cleansing breath in through your nose, hold it for a moment, and exhale slowly through your mouth. Repeat this process a few times for each area of tension to release stress.

- *Identify your primary and secondary nourishment.* Use your journal or a pad of paper to make a list of all the ways you receive nourishment.

  › Divide the page into two columns. Write "primary nourishment" at the top of one column and "secondary nourishment" at the top of the other.

  › Under the primary nourishment heading, list the relationships, as well as the social activities, events, and practices that help you manage your stress load. Who and what is truly nourishing for you?

  › Under the secondary nourishment heading, list the ways you receive secondary nourishment. For example, specific meals or food items; time in nature; movement practices; or an item of comfort in your home, such as a weighted blanket or cozy spot. I often do this activity with my clients in session, and sometimes it brings aha moments when they realize they aren't as limited on helpful resources as they thought.

  › Take a picture of your lists or type the items into the notes app of your phone. Refer to them when you feel overwhelmed by stress. Your lists provide great answers for when you ask yourself, *How can I nourish myself right now?*

3

HOW YOUR SELF-TALK IMPACTS YOUR HEALTH

"Are you ready to talk about your test results?" I asked my client Selena. She nodded emphatically as I slid my laptop over for her to view the screen. Selena had sought out my nutrition coaching services for her digestive issues.

"I've tried everything," she told me in our first appointment. "I've tried eliminating foods, but I can't tell a difference. I went to a GI doctor who said it was IBS but never really told me what was causing it. I take some of the pills he told me to take, but I don't notice a difference with those either. I tried probiotics—nothing. I'm so uncomfortable with my bloated belly. Now my skin is breaking out with these weird patches, and I'm wondering if that's connected too."

As I listened to Selena share more of her story, the puzzle pieces came together. She had struggled with an eating disorder in college, but it was mostly under control now. However, she was still hypercritical about her appearance, so much so that she asked friends not to tag her on social media without first getting her approval.

"I know I sound crazy," she said. "And sometimes I feel crazy. But I only like certain angles of myself in pictures. It relieves my anxiety if I'm only tagged in pictures that I like."

By the time we got the results of her GI-MAP test, a stool test that analyzes gut microbial composition, I wasn't surprised by the results. I pointed to a marker on the screen, secretory IgA.[1]

"By any chance, do you tend to struggle with chronic negative self-talk, like a pretty loud inner critic?" I asked.

Selena stared at me in awe. "Pretty much every day. How did you know?"

I smiled at her reassuringly. "Because low levels of this marker are often associated with anger and frustration, and it tends to be low in my clients who are negative with themselves."[2]

Your Body Responds to Your Thoughts

Have you ever considered that negative self-talk might be a chronic stressor in your life? Maybe you don't think of it that way and believe that your inner critic is a good thing, or even a friend who motivates you to keep going. She reminds you not to miss appointments, to wake up on time (without hitting snooze), and to say no to the second brownie.

But she's typically not very nice about it. She sounds more like a drill sergeant than a friend. And every cell in your body listens to her tone. When the tone is negative, your body considers the inner critic a threat. And remember, your body knows how to respond to threats. What your brain perceives as true—that you are facing a threat—creates a cascade of biochemical signals that contribute to more stress and dysfunction.

If you allow your inner critic to run the show with negativity and toxic self-talk, your cells pick up on that. In his book *The Biology of Belief*, cell biologist Bruce Lipton writes, "When we change the way we perceive the world, that is, when we 'change our beliefs,' we change the blood's neurochemical composition, which then initiates a complementary change in the body's cells."[3] In other words, your interpretation of the world makes an imprint on your biology.

One of the clearest examples of how your thoughts affect the function of your body is the hypothalamic-pituitary-adrenal axis (HPA). The HPA axis is a communication system between three organs—the hypothalamus, pituitary gland, and adrenal glands—and is crucial for your body's stress management.[4]

When the emotional sensor of the brain (the amygdala) senses a threat, it initiates the HPA axis by sending a signal to the *hypothalamus*. The hypothalamus passes the signal along to the *pituitary gland* to activate the release of stress hormones. These stress hormones, such as cortisol, are produced in the *adrenal glands*, which sit on top of the kidneys. Cortisol sounds the alarm to get blood pumping faster, slow digestion, increase blood sugar, mess with the thyroid a little, and impact reproductive hormones and even the immune system. The goal is to prepare the body to face a short-term threat. However, at the brain level, when stress goes on too long or too many threats happen at once, the amygdala (the emotional response center of the brain) can become overactive.

When an overactive amygdala continues to hit the panic button, the HPA axis continues to release stress hormones, which leads to hypervigilance, anxiety, and that jumpy feeling—all of which create more stress. But most importantly, all those stress hormones make it impossible for the prefrontal cortex to activate. The prefrontal cortex is the mature part of your brain responsible for rational thought. However, when you're facing a threat, the amygdala fails to connect to the prefrontal cortex, taking it "offline." That's why you find it hard to focus, make decisions, control impulses, and even show empathy to others when you're stressed—the part of your brain that does those things is deactivated.

Now, remember what I told you about how a lack of nutrients creates physiological stress? If a perceived threat triggers the release of cortisol, slowing digestion, and if your body is so stressed it's depleted of nutrients needed to create feel-good chemicals—such as serotonin, GABA, and dopamine—your body is not getting signals that you're happy and safe. Your chemicals get thrown out of whack, and then you experience all kinds of mood disruptions at an even more extreme level. All because of a perceived threat.

We see this same cascading effect play out in many areas of the body. Sometimes, rather than using the term *HPA axis*, experts will refer to this network of communication as the hypothalamic-pituitary-adrenal-thyroid-gonadal (HPATG) axis. That's because your thyroid and gonadal (reproductive) system are also in cahoots with your thoughts, waiting to adjust their functioning based on the signals they receive. As neuroscientist Wendy Suzuki states, this chronic response to stress "affects our brains and bodies in numerous ways, at numerous levels, including the neuroendocrine system, the autonomic nervous system, and the cardiovascular and immune systems."[5] Which means every bodily system listens to your thoughts.

This is how your body is meant to function. *God designed you with an internal alert system that is highly functioning, highly protective, and highly sensitive to your thoughts.* He created this system to work on a loop, so your cells respond to your thoughts and your thoughts respond back to your cells. Your body and brain are intricately connected and sensitive to each other's signals. Your thoughts affect how you feel. They create messages that impact every system in your body. This is a good thing—a human thing! But this feedback loop can also have some dramatic consequences if you're not paying attention—especially if your inner critic runs the show.

Repetitive Negativity Is a Trap

Repetitive negativity is a chronic stressor, but it's an incredibly adaptive response when you're in survival mode. Your brain is always scanning for danger, looking to protect you, and when it encounters familiar territory such as repetitive negative thinking, it will keep on keeping on, perpetuating negative thought patterns. This is often referred to as the negativity bias.[6] The negativity bias is a natural preference our brains give to negative experiences, emotions, and memories over positive ones. This negativity bias is why we tend to be more activated by negative information, and why we fixate on distressing events and conversations more than positive ones.

If you think about it, this is an incredible tool for protection—at first glance. A bias for dwelling on the negative keeps us alert to important or life-threatening events that need our attention. As trauma researcher Bessel van der Kolk states, "The most important job of the brain is to ensure our survival, even under the most miserable conditions. Everything else is secondary."[7]

However, when that negativity bias becomes an entrenched pattern of negative self-talk that draws you inward and away from the truth of your God-given identity, it's a trap—one that creates a vicious cycle of stress. And because it's a stressor, it can lead to negative consequences—for both your health and your ability to receive primary nourishment.

Negativity Is a Trap for Your Health

The health trap occurs when our patterns of negative self-talk lead to negative outcomes with our physical health. My client Selena is a good example. Because she struggled with a chronic loop of fear and frustration about her appearance, it's no surprise that she also struggled with chronic gut issues. The trap for Selena was that her inner critic made her gut symptoms worse, and her gut symptoms made her feel worse about herself. She was trapped in a vicious cycle and wasn't sure how to stop it.

We've already identified the HPA axis as one way we can trace the body's response to negative thoughts, but it isn't the only way. Recent research into the *gut-brain axis* and *psychoneuroimmunology* helps demonstrate how repetitive negativity impacts our physical health.

The gut-brain axis. The gut-brain axis is a bidirectional communication network that involves (yep, you guessed it) your brain and your gut. When I refer to your gut, I'm talking about the entire gastrointestinal tract, a twenty-five to thirty-foot tunnel that works as an exchange corridor, transmitting and receiving information.

The gut and brain are connected via the vagus nerve that involves the enteric nervous system (the nervous system of the gastrointestinal tract). The enteric nervous system contains one hundred million to five hundred million neurons, which is the largest collection of nerve cells in the body, aside from the brain. The vagus nerve starts at the base of your skull and connects to your throat, heart, blood vessels, gallbladder, liver, and intestines. But what happens in the vagus nerve doesn't stay in the vagus nerve. You've probably felt it doing its communication work. Ever had a "gut feeling"? Ever gotten butterflies before speaking in front of a group of people? That's your brain sending signals to your gut. However, 90 percent of the nerve fibers are *afferent*, meaning the communication travels from gut to brain. So your gut may be talking to your brain *more* than your brain talks to your gut.

Our gut microbiome is the ecosystem of bacteria, viruses, and fungi housed in our digestive system. These microbes modulate our mood. In fact, over 90 percent of our "happy" neurotransmitter serotonin is created by the gut microbiome. Our microbiome also shapes our metabolism, digestion, satiety, pain response, food preferences and cravings, and even our stress levels.

The microbes in our gut must be balanced, or we can experience unpleasant symptoms, such as indigestion, bloating, skin rashes, inflammation, joint pain, food sensitivities, chronic fatigue, and many others. This imbalance of microbes is often referred to as *dysbiosis*. While stress can alter our microbial composition, an altered microbial composition can also decrease our ability to manage stress. It's extremely cyclical and, of course, begs the chicken-and-egg question for many of us struggling with mood disorders: *Are my microbes causing me to suffer, or is my suffering disrupting my microbes?* And for those struggling with mental distress and gut distress, this cycle makes it difficult to know where to start the healing process—whether with the gut or the brain.

Psychoneuroimmunology. Psychoneuroimmunology is a new field of study focused on the communication network that involves your central nervous system (your brain, spinal cord, and neurons) and your immune system. For many years, scientists believed that the brain and the immune system were separate. The study of psychoneuroimmunology, also referred to as psychoneuroimmunoendocrinology, explores how the brain and the immune system are interconnected and signal one another.

Your immune system uses proteins called cytokines to communicate with your brain. And your brain plays a major role in how those proteins are formed. Neuropeptides, also referred to as the "molecules of emotion," are chains of amino acids that are believed to be formed by emotions that originate in the brain. In response to different types of stress, neuropeptides can signal inflammatory cytokine production in the body, which is immune-protective in the short-term but can wreak havoc and bring more distress to the body in the long-term. One study showed that social stress releases a completely different kind of cytokine than physical stress.[8] Negative emotions also trigger the immune system to secrete pro-inflammatory cytokines. For example, fear can trigger IL-6, another type of inflammatory cytokine.[9] How crazy is that? Your emotions communicate with your immune system!

Microglia are considered the immune cells of the brain. When the body's immune system is overactivated, the brain can respond by sending out overactivated microglia to launch an attack on brain synapses and increase inflammation. As science journalist Donna Jackson Nakazawa explains,

> It's all one system, connected by a brain-immune superhighway, and when the body is overwhelmed, the brain can become overwhelmed too. The same environmental toxins, chemicals, and processed food diets that are catalysts for disease in the body can trigger microglia to launch an immune attack against the brain.[10]

I won't quiz you on the science (I promise), but remember this: Your thoughts trigger a cascade of responses from your immune system, and its purpose is to protect you.

One missing puzzle piece in my bipolar diagnosis at age eighteen is the fact that I was also diagnosed with mononucleosis at the same time. Could it be that my overactive immune system was fighting so hard to defeat the mono that it targeted my brain, leading to a manic episode? I'll never know for sure, but psychoneuroimmunology gives me hope that other people in my situation will receive more comprehensive treatment than I did.

I know we've covered a lot of hard science, so allow me to recap. Your thoughts are made from your perception of the world. That perception (based on truth or not) sends signals in various ways to the chemical messengers or systems in your body that run the show on just about everything else. And therein lies the trap: When you constantly criticize yourself and beat yourself up, you create more stress inside your body, and out of protection, your body alters its important functions to survive the stressor, which may unfortunately create more mental stress.

Negativity Is a Trap for Your Primary Nourishment

The bullies in your brain, the lies you believe, and the old repetitive sound clips that pop up from time to time are not lifegiving. The negativity prevents you from living out your purpose and engaging with your primary nourishment—foundational relationships with God, others, and yourself—in healthy ways. It keeps you from seeing yourself the way your heavenly Father sees you.

Negative self-talk promotes conformity to a culture that determines worth based on transitory things, such as achievements and appearance. But you're created for and called to something better. The apostle Paul writes, "Don't copy the behavior and customs of this world, but let God transform you into a new person by changing the way you think" (Romans 12:2, NLT). He also says, "To set the mind on the flesh is death, but to set the mind on the Spirit is life and peace" (Romans 8:6).

Negative self-talk is adaptive and protective in the same way that gut dysbiosis and immune hypervigilance are. But we must stop the vicious cycle—the lies and the internal negativity—that too often prevents us from taking steps toward renewal and healing.

Negative self-talk triggers that trap:

See? It happened again. You're never going to be good enough.
You can't do anything right.
You are the laziest person you know.
Nobody wants to talk to you. You always say the dumbest things.

You're the only one who has this issue. Everyone else is fine. You'll never be able to recover from this.

Such self-talk can eventually lead to isolation. Even if you aren't intentionally cutting yourself off from others or actively harming yourself, you can easily turn inward and not allow yourself to receive primary nourishment of any kind. Perhaps you're married, but you can't bear to be touched by your husband or become intimate in any way. Maybe you want to have deeper friendships, but you are too afraid to reach out for fear of being rejected. Maybe you've been diagnosed with a mental illness, and you feel like you'll never again feel regulated or "normal." Or perhaps you want to do something nice for yourself, such as learn to cook with more vegetables, go for a daily walk, or practice meditation, but you can't add anything more to your schedule because it's filled up by your need to avoid and suppress. That familiar negativity keeps you trapped and isolated from the primary nourishment you need most.

When you're constantly beating yourself up, you'll struggle to see yourself the way God sees you. You'll find it difficult to receive care from others. And you'll find it nearly impossible to give yourself grace and compassion.

If you struggle with negative self-talk, you know the solution isn't as simple as telling yourself to snap out of it. You can't passively bypass yourself by "letting go and letting God." Escaping the trap requires active engagement as you rewire the way you think. And it starts with mindfulness.

Mindfulness Matters

One of the greatest tools I've discovered on my own journey to healing from negative self-talk is mindfulness. To practice mindfulness is to pause and step outside your dominant thoughts so you can observe them. You investigate by becoming an observer or scientist of your own experience.

When I observe my negative thoughts, I can acknowledge that I have a self-defeating behavior but do so without simultaneously berating myself for it. When I allow myself to be curious rather than judgmental about my negative thoughts, I open myself up to respond with self-compassion rather than self-condemnation.

Remember how surprised my client Selena was when we looked at her test results and I asked whether she struggled with negative self-talk? Her decreased levels of secretory IgA—antibodies in the intestinal lining—indicated that her thoughts and emotions were taking a toll on her body. I knew this because studies have demonstrated that anger and frustration can lead to decreased protective levels of secretory IgA in our digestive tract. However, those

Stop the Downward Spiral

When you practice mindfulness by observing your self-talk, you can pause and redirect your thoughts to stop the downward spiral. Here are some examples of how to do that:

Instead of, *I can't believe I'm thinking these negative thoughts again!*

You can say, *It's really interesting that these thoughts came up again. I wonder what triggered them. Maybe I'm experiencing more stress than I thought, and I need to do something nourishing for myself.*

Instead of, *I hate the way I look in pictures!*

You can say, *I'm feeling insecure right now, and old wounds are resurfacing. I thought I healed those, but it looks like I am still hurting deep down.*

Instead of, *What is wrong with me for thinking these thoughts?*

You can say, *I am being mean to myself. I wonder what caused that? Maybe I can talk to someone about this so I don't stay stuck in my mind for too long.*

same studies also demonstrated that care and compassion *increase* levels of secretory IgA.[11] Practicing mindfulness helps us create compassion that is transformative, even on an immune system level! That's because mindfulness interrupts the stress response. Practicing mindfulness has also been shown to decrease the size of the amygdala, the sometimes-overemotional responder in the brain that tells your hypothalamus to panic.[12]

Mindful awareness is a helpful way to observe your thoughts and the role they play in your behaviors. But don't stop with observing; it's only the first step. The next step is to identify the lies in your negative self-talk and replace them with truth.

Consume the Truth

There's a common saying in the world of neuroscience: "Neurons that fire together, wire together."[13] This refers to the idea that the brain thrives on repetition and creates connections based on information that is familiar. Go back to the negativity bias: If your negative self-talk is familiar to the brain, it will become increasingly repetitive, and it will look like truth—even when it's not. That's the bad news.

Here's the good news: Thanks to what we know of neuroplasticity, the brain's ability to adapt and change, you can rewire the entire system. To rewire the system, begin by looking at your current patterns of consumption. What are you consuming that causes you to ruminate on the negative, encouraging repetitive, self-critical thought patterns? Specifically, what do you routinely read, watch, scroll through, and listen to? Then consider whether what you're consuming is causing you to believe a lie.

As an adolescent, I frequently consumed celebrity gossip magazines, loving it when they shared their secrets to being thin. I overdosed on diet articles and books, waiting for that one thing to bring me lasting satisfaction in my body. I ate up relationship advice, flirting techniques, and ways to set goals to achieve all my heart's desires. The common denominator in all that mental food was one thing. *Me.* I chose to believe *I* held the key to unlocking my own happiness and success.

That pattern of consumption led me to buy into the lie that if I didn't take charge, no one would. The combination of past trauma with an overachieving personality led me to believe that not even God could support me in my dreams. I needed to make them happen myself.

Self-criticism danced with self-inflation. When I wasn't beating myself up, I was checking off items on my mental to-do list to appear farther ahead—to prove to myself that I wasn't as bad as I thought I was, that my brain wasn't as broken as they told me.

When I based my self-help strategy on what I alone could do, I no longer needed a Savior, because that savior was me. The dangerous lie of self-saving created a wall between me and God. The problem was that I never quite measured up to the standards I set for myself. I needed to be filled with truth, but I was burdened by a Jenga tower of negativity and the lies that held it all together.

The narrative we buy into will look different for everyone. For me, it was the lie that I could be my own savior. For you, the lie may be that you're only as good as the image you present, that taking care of your own needs is selfish, or that you must be a certain size to be healthy or attractive. The only way to kill lies like these is to starve them by consuming truth alone. Trust me, if self-effort could have saved anyone from the tyranny of negative self-talk, I would have found the three-step plan in a magazine and saved myself a long time ago. But it's almost impossible to start believing truth when lies and negativity are all you've known.

So how do you let Jesus, who is *the* Truth, into your healing process?

You listen.

You listen to his words by reading his Word—by saturating your mind with truth.

There is no substitute for God's Word. This book isn't. A daily devotional or Christian podcast isn't. A Sunday sermon isn't. Worship music isn't. Scripture itself proclaims, "The word of God is alive and powerful" (Hebrews 4:12, NLT). When the truth of God's Word begins to replace your lies and toxic thoughts, it creates positive downstream effects in every area of your life. When you are overconsuming the truth and starving the twisty lies, that is when true renewal of the mind begins.

MAKING THE MIND-BODY CONNECTION

Choose one or more of the following practices to help you begin to observe your thoughts. Try to engage with these activities without judgment. If you don't feel ready to practice any of them right now, notice that with self-compassion too.

- *Practice mindfulness.* Find a quiet place where you won't be distracted and sit in a comfortable position—legs uncrossed, hands resting lightly on your thighs or lap, and back straight. Take a few deep breaths, in through your nose and out through your mouth, noticing the silence apart from your breathing. Observe your thoughts. What do you notice? If your thoughts seem scattered, notice that. If you're thinking, *I don't want to sit still,* notice that. Maybe you're not really thinking anything particular; that's okay too. Simply take note of what happens when you sit still, doing nothing. If a dominant thought pops up, let it pass through your mind like clouds passing across a blue sky. Continue to practice stillness, allowing nothing to distract you. It's okay if doing so feels strange, especially at first. Simply observe that in a nonjudgmental way as well.

HOW YOUR SELF-TALK IMPACTS YOUR HEALTH

- ***Take notes on your negative thoughts.*** Choose one day this week to observe your negative thoughts. Use your journal, a pad of paper, or the notes app on your phone to document the negative thoughts you have about yourself or your situation. If you have one thought multiple times, make a tally mark next to it on your list. At the end of the day, review your list and consider how much of your day was taken up by negative self-talk. The more aware you are of your negative thought patterns, the more equipped you'll be to replace those lies with truth.

- ***Crowd in truth.*** Listen to God's thoughts about you by spending time in Scripture. Set aside time every day for the next seven days to reflect on a verse or a passage of Scripture that tells you what God thinks of you. If you're concerned this might take up too much time, I have an option for you. I love the concept of "morning minutes." Take three minutes in the morning (yes, just three minutes) to prayerfully read a verse or passage that affirms how God sees you. Write down the verse or a word or phrase that stands out to you on a sticky note and post it where you will see it throughout the day. Here are some options to get you started:

  › Psalm 139:13-16

  › Romans 8:14-15

  › Psalm 23

  › Galatians 4:6-7

  › 1 Samuel 16:7

  › 2 Corinthians 5:17

4

COULD YOUR PESKY THOUGHTS BE PROTECTIVE?

When my daughter was recently sick with nasal congestion, she passed through our living room, snotting into a tissue, and said, "I better not get kidnapped now."

I laughed and immediately responded, "That's exactly what I think when I'm sick too!"

Thanks to crime television and movies, I have an irrational fear of my mouth being duct-taped shut when I'm congested. I would stop breathing. I wouldn't survive. I felt so validated that someone else experienced this same type of irrational fear.

What about you? Do you experience any anxiety flickers you think might sound crazy if you were to speak them out loud? I asked my Instagram followers the same question. Here is a sample of their responses:

"I'm afraid to go on a group tour, because what if I need to use the bathroom and I can't get to one in time, or we can't stop?"

"When I go to the dentist and I'm getting my teeth cleaned, I'm paranoid they'll drop a tool down my throat."

"Every time I open the washer or dryer, I think I'm going to find a snake in there."

"When I'm standing at the top of a tall structure, building, or mountain, I wonder what would happen if I accidentally fell. Or what if I lost my footing and went forward? Or what if because I'm thinking about falling, I make myself fall?"

This next one is my favorite because I totally think this too:

"Sometimes I'm afraid to get up and use the bathroom in a public gathering like a church service because I wonder, *What would happen if I started doing cartwheels right now?* Then, *Uh-oh, now my brain is thinking about cartwheels. What if my body does the cartwheels even though I don't want to do the cartwheels?*"

Chances are these pesky thoughts don't last long in your brain. They aren't obsessive or intrusive at a diagnostic level. But they show up like a game of Whack-A-Mole, don't they? They especially like to visit in the middle of the night, on nights when sleep is interrupted due to overly stressful seasons. That's when the brain goes wild, creating new stories and plot twists, some so ridiculous that you wake up in the morning and wonder what in the world you were thinking.

Everyone experiences thought patterns like these at some point. Usually, they are benign and not a reason to seek support. My daughter doesn't barricade herself in her room when she's sick to avoid being kidnapped; my friend doesn't stop washing her clothes due to her snake fear. I affectionately refer to these pesky thoughts

COULD YOUR PESKY THOUGHTS BE PROTECTIVE?

as "WCSB," or "Worst-Case Scenario Brain." They are typically not limiting and don't deter us from taking part in everyday life. But on the flip side of WCSB is another form of overthinking. When things are going *too* well, we anticipate something bad will soon happen. When left unchecked, this type of anxious anticipation can become problematic or hinder functioning.

I experienced this kind of overthinking consistently throughout my first year of marriage. I got married at twenty-eight as a single mom with a five-year-old daughter. While I was wise and mature in some ways, in many other ways I was haunted by shame. My past, especially through college, had been marked by bad decisions caused by mania, medication, alcohol, and just plain self-destructiveness. At one point I stopped caring and just let life happen to me until, thankfully, the birth of my daughter snapped me out of my downward spiral.

Early in my marriage, I harbored doubts that my husband could truly accept me and love me—despite my past and my bipolar diagnosis. So I lived in fear, waiting for something bad to happen. With every conflict (and of course, there were conflicts—usually about sex, money, or co-parenting a kindergartner), I believed he'd be better off if he hadn't married me. Maybe I was too broken for him. And maybe it was only a matter of time until he came to the same conclusion.

My constant overthinking, WCSB, and disaster scouting bounced around in my brain like a high-speed ping-pong match, and I believed my big feelings and loud thoughts would be too much for anyone, much less for someone who hadn't experienced the kind of struggles I had. These thoughts weighed me down and only created more conflict in my marriage, until I decided to address them. What I didn't realize was that my brain had a good reason for overthinking and spinning out worst-case scenarios. It was trying to protect me.

There Are Good Reasons We Overthink

Believe it or not, overthinking is part of our design. It's an alert system that prepares us to be on guard for any scenario that threatens our survival. When we overthink, we are trying to keep ourselves safe, and there are at least four reasons we do so: to protect, to prepare, to control, and to avoid feeling.

We Overthink to Protect

Everyone develops different protective responses throughout their lives. Your protective responses are unique to you. They are what keep you safe. If you've experienced the imprint of trauma, your protective responses serve to make sure you don't get caught off guard again. Protective responses only become problematic when they make it difficult for you to show up in the world as your genuine self or when they become debilitating in some way.

To understand how our brains use overthinking to protect us, we need to understand the autonomic nervous system. As part of the body's command center, the autonomic nervous system controls involuntary bodily functions, such as heart rate, breathing, and pupil dilation. The two main divisions of the autonomic nervous system are the sympathetic state and the parasympathetic state.

> *Sympathetic state*: Commonly known as the fight-flight-freeze response, this state is activated when the body (through the HPA axis) detects a real or perceived threat.
>
> *Parasympathetic state*: This state is activated when the HPA axis feels safe, calm, and regulated. It's also known as the rest-and-digest state because it allows the body to utilize all available nutrients to repair and heal.

COULD YOUR PESKY THOUGHTS BE PROTECTIVE?

Our bodies are designed to live in balance, also known as homeostasis. We're designed to adapt to all kinds of stressors, both emotional and physiological. The beauty of the sympathetic and parasympathetic states is that they keep everything in homeostasis to protect us.

Although both states are essential, we often hear that it's somehow bad to be in a fight, flight, or freeze state. What most people don't realize is that this is how we get things done. For example, a little bit of sympathetic activation helps us to meet deadlines or act quickly when there is an emergency. With a helpful boost of norepinephrine and adrenaline, our thinking gets clearer for a short period. The body wants us to survive these temporary threats to our survival, so it does what it always does when it detects danger. The key word there is *temporary*.

We don't want to stay in a sympathetic state for too long. When the body gets trapped in a sympathetic state, it leads to a *hyperadrenal* state of chronic stress, activating a fight-or-flight response. The *hyper* in *hyperadrenal* means the adrenal glands are *over*producing stress hormones, which can lead to health issues such as insomnia, hypertension, rapid heart rate, high blood sugar, weakened immune function, and electrolyte imbalances. Symptoms we might experience in this state include shaking, racing heart, anxiety, inability to take a deep breath, fear, or a need to move.

When we get too overwhelmed by whatever the threat may be, the body activates the freeze response. This is an extreme *hypoadrenal* state. The *hypo* in *hypoadrenal* means the adrenal glands are *under*producing stress hormones. Out of protection, the body lowers its cortisol production, which causes us to feel completely depleted, with no reserves. This often happens when we've lived in a state of high cortisol for so long that the body—in its intelligent design—chooses to use the minimum amount of energy to function. Emotional symptoms we might experience in this state include exhaustion (especially upon waking), low motivation, or disassociation, all of which can look a lot like depression. Physical symptoms can show up as hypotension, low blood sugar, low heart rate, autoimmunity, hypothyroidism, lethargy, and electrolyte imbalances. Perhaps the simplest way to think of the freeze response under intense stress is that it feels like the body has chosen to play possum as a form of self-protection.

In recent years, another response of the sympathetic nervous system has been identified—the fawn response, which is also known as the "tend-and-befriend" response. The fawn response is an attempt to minimize danger by appeasing the threat. It might involve behaviors such as excessive caretaking or controlling our environment as a strategy to protect ourselves—and everyone else—from an oncoming threat. For example, this might look like having difficulty saying no or trying to avoid conflict by agreeing with others' opinions even when we secretly disagree. Or it might look like pouring all our time and energy into managing the family calendar and kids' activities and being the perfect homemaker because our protective brains rationalize that if we don't, our world might fall apart. For many of my clients, it's easier to tend to the needs and emotions of others than it is to tend to their own. Fawning is a way to respond to internal stress without having to deal with unpleasant emotions. However, it's still depleting and takes a toll on the body.

Ideally, we want to be in the parasympathetic state of safety and calm for considerably longer than the sympathetic states of fight, flight, freeze, and fawn. Unfortunately, too many of us end up in a chronic sympathetic state that impacts our mental function. For example, in a chronic sympathetic state we might forget things or experience brain fog, which activates the inner critic who tells us we're messing up. Our anxiety increases because, what if the brain fog causes us to miss something? The anxiety then leads to chronic hypervigilance as we try to protect ourselves by staying alert to any potential danger, real or imagined. And the sympathetic activation cycle continues.

The good news in all of this is that your body and brain are always on your side, always trying to protect you and alert you when something is wrong. Your job is to listen to what your body and brain are telling you so you can make changes when necessary. For example, when you're experiencing a state of overthinking, you can listen to your brain by asking a quick check-in question: "Do these thoughts I'm having serve a purpose of protection right now?" If so, a follow-up question could be, "What do my thoughts tell me about the state of my safety?" This is a real-time way to practice mindfulness and offer yourself compassion. If all else fails to help restore your mind to calm, use the "that's interesting" statement. For example, "That's interesting. I'm feeling super anxious right now. I wonder what is causing that." Being a compassionate observer of your thoughts helps give you some distance and safety from the thoughts themselves.

The fight, flight, freeze, and fawn responses are perfect examples of protective responses that occur when we're in a sympathetic-activated state of overthinking. These responses help us adapt to increased stress levels. But protection is only one reason we overthink.

We Overthink to Prepare

I've decided that there should be one more beatitude in the Bible: "Blessed are the overthinkers, for they shall be prepared for any situation." When you overthink to prepare, it means you are alert and ready for anything. Mentally and emotionally, symptoms of overthinking to prepare may look like chronic anxiety, intrusive thoughts, and putting up walls or not trusting people even when they have proven they are trustworthy. Physical symptoms might include high blood pressure, severe digestive issues, or difficulty taking a deep breath when stressed. Overthinking to prepare puts your body in "fight" mode so you're ready for any kind of threat, thanks to the signals from your brain.

The need to feel prepared often comes from having felt previously caught off guard by an unwanted and unpleasant experience. You cope with your fears that this might happen again by rehearsing all the what-ifs so you're ready to respond to any potential bad scenario. This is the WCSB in action. Maybe you wake up at 3:00 a.m., your mind racing about a situation at work. So you run through all kinds of scenarios in your head. You prepare speeches so you'll have a ready response for the difficult coworker or the demanding boss, anticipating conflicts that haven't even happened yet. And then you run through all the scenarios again and your mind is caught in a loop that is almost impossible to escape, which makes it impossible to go back to sleep.

A great analogy for overthinking to be prepared is how my dog, Luka, shadows me. Luka is a goldendoodle, meaning he's part poodle and part golden retriever. The extreme loyalty he gets from the golden retriever side of his family tree is evident in his need to always be with me—because his biggest fear (aside from fireworks on the Fourth of July) is *not* being with me. As I write this, he's on the floor next to me, sleeping peacefully. However, if at any moment I move my chair back, he will immediately hop up, ready to follow me to wherever I go next. He is so prepared to mimic my movements, he can't even tend to his own napping needs.

If life has primed you to prepare for the worst, your brain and body are as focused on scanning for potential threats as Luka is focused on scanning for my potential movement. When your brain senses a threat, your body prepares for action, often at the expense of restful sleep and other basic human needs, such as digestion. Running through preparedness options may give you some measure of temporary relief, but over time, chronic overthinking will become oppressive and take a toll on your body.

We Overthink to Control

Overthinking gives us the illusion of control. We reason that if we think through every possible outcome, we can ensure that nothing that bad happens. Makes sense, right? Nothing bad ever happens when we predict it and plan for it. So if we analyze all the possible outcomes, we ensure we are in control and won't be thrown off course if the inevitable bad thing does happen.

Just as with overthinking to prepare, overthinking to control is often a response to past experience. Maybe you forgot your child's medication once on a trip, and now every time you go on vacation, you check, double-check, and triple-check to make sure you have not just the medication but everything else you might potentially need. This can be super helpful if you're going on a trip, but it can become overwhelming when it develops into an obsessive need to have it all together that constantly plagues your brain.

I often see this need to control when addressing my clients' relationships with food. Some people tend to get more fearful of food if they're afraid their bodies will have a negative response to it. The term for this is *orthorexia*, a disorder in which one is obsessed with eating only food that is healthy. Orthorexia is often rooted in a fear that a person's health issues won't be healed unless they have a perfect diet. They have a deep need to control their health condition through strict adherence to eating only what they believe is "clean." At its worst, this need to control food intake dominates every thought, to the point that it interferes with enjoyment at social gatherings or casual outings with friends. To the person suffering, maintaining a healthy diet may have started out of good intent, to support the health of their body. But with an overthinking brain, it turned into an obsessive need for control.

We Overthink to Avoid Feeling

Overthinking can be a way to avoid difficult feelings. Don't want to dwell on anxiety or other confusing emotions? No problem! Just jump into an overthinking rabbit hole. For example, if I'm feeling anxious about something, I can distract myself from the anxiety by thinking about something else. I might spend hours on Google researching a topic that interests me, or doomscroll social media, or obsess over an innocuous comment my husband made recently *(Maybe he really didn't like the chicken and only said he did to avoid offending me)*. It doesn't matter what the issue is as long as it keeps me from having to dig into what my real feelings are, or why I am experiencing those feelings to begin with. This version of overthinking distracts me from addressing the unpleasant feeling at the root. But suppressing the feeling often creates additional issues, such as picking fights with my spouse over his comments about my chicken. When this happens, I unintentionally create a conflict that didn't exist before, all to avoid addressing what's *really* going on. At its worst, avoidance overthinking creates a spiral—a mental tornado that rips through the landscape, leaving a trail of destruction in its wake. There's no stopping to reason with it; it just barrels through.

Ironically, this unstoppable spiral may initially feel stress-relieving, thanks to the familiar hit of stress chemicals such as adrenaline. Like other forms of overthinking, it is a survival response, and if this is a go-to strategy for you, it has likely served you as a coping mechanism for many years.

Yes, the brain has several good reasons for overthinking. But when overthinking becomes chronic, it creates a sympathetic state in the body. And if you don't remember anything else about the sympathetic state of the body, remember this: *Your body can't heal in a sympathetic-dominated state.* Your body can only find optimal healing when it's in a parasympathetic rest-and-digest state.

Also remember that our bodies are always on our side, always trying to protect us and always trying to alert us when something is wrong. When we understand that our patterns of thought are intended to serve and protect us, we can tune in to their alerts without being debilitated by them and change course when necessary.

Protective Alerts in the Storm

One of my favorite gospel stories comes from Mark 4, when a storm arises as Jesus and the disciples are crossing a lake in a boat.

> A furious squall came up, and the waves broke over the boat, so that it was nearly swamped. Jesus was in the stern, sleeping on a cushion. The disciples woke him and said to him, "Teacher, don't you care if we drown?"
> He got up, rebuked the wind and said to the waves, "Quiet! Be still!" Then the wind died down and it was completely calm.
> MARK 4:37-39, NIV

While the disciples panicked, likely thinking of every worst-case scenario possible, Jesus was asleep on a cushion, clearly unbothered. And when the disciples woke him up, Jesus told the storm to stop. And it did! The wind calmed down, and everything went back to normal.

What stands out to me most about this scene is not the fact that Jesus calmed the storm, though that is amazing. What stands out is that he was right there with the disciples, and yet they still panicked. Even though they'd seen Jesus perform all kinds of miracles and truly believed he was the Son of God, they still feared the worst-case scenario. In their momentary panic, their survival brains eclipsed their rational brains, and they were convinced they wouldn't make it. Sound familiar?

Those of us who have struggled with our mental health for most of our lives—especially those of us who have the diagnoses and the meds and the therapy bills to show for it—understand this dynamic on a deeply painful level.

When I first struggled with depression and racing thoughts in my teens, I thought I was a bad Christian. I thought I needed to pray harder. I thought I didn't have enough faith. I remember sitting in church listening to worship music and trying to pray but feeling stuck. *Why doesn't God hear me? Doesn't he see what I'm struggling with? Why won't he heal me and fix me? It must be a sin issue.* I was doing everything I knew to get better, but I still couldn't get him to calm the storm.

It would take many years for me to see that, despite my stormy seas, he was in the boat with me. I didn't realize it at the time, but he was already at work through my body to alert me to danger through my nervous system fluctuation. He was already at work through the people who supported me during the darkest times. He was already at work through the protection I received even during times of self-destruction. I couldn't see it then, but I see it now. He was with me through all the storms.

Know this: Jesus is in the boat with you—even if you think he's sleeping on the job. Even if you think he's left you. Even if your brain is so foggy from overthinking that you don't know how to pray. He's there, and he knows.

He has designed you with a body that is scanning the world around you to alert you to danger, and sometimes those scans come with unpleasant symptoms such as anxiety, racing thoughts, intrusive reminders, and repetitive patterns of negative thinking.

When you learn to tune in to what your nervous system is telling you and lean into this protection, you can stay ahead of the storm. You can engage mindfully with your thoughts rather than be held hostage by them. Instead of looking at the storm in fear and panic, you can look to the one who calms it.

MAKING THE MIND-BODY CONNECTION

A breath prayer is a type of prayer that matches the words of Scripture to the inhale-exhale rhythm of breathing. By praying a few words while inhaling, and a few words while exhaling, mind and body connect as breath becomes prayer.

I often use a prayer from the book *Breath as Prayer* by Jennifer Tucker, which draws on the following verse: "He stilled the storm to a whisper, and the waves of the sea were hushed" (Psalm 107:29, CSB). As you take a deep inhale through your nose, pray, "You still the storms to a whisper." Then exhale as you pray, "You hush the waves of the sea."[1] Repeat the prayer three to five times, inhaling and exhaling with each phrase. Notice how you feel before, during, and after prayer.

You might also try it with other phrases of Scripture. For example, the most ancient form of the prayer dates to the third century and draws on the biblical story of a blind man named Bartimaeus, who called out, "Jesus, Son of David, have mercy on me!" (Mark 10:47, NLT). While inhaling slowly, pray, "Jesus Christ, Son of God"; and while exhaling slowly, "have mercy on me." Or, from Psalm 62:1 (NIV), "My soul finds rest" (inhale), "in God alone" (exhale). Or, from Psalm 46:10, "Be still, and know" (inhale), "that I am God" (exhale). Use your breath prayer throughout the day anytime you need to calm your mind and be reminded of God's love and care for you.

5

YOUR BREATH REFLECTS YOUR STRESS LEVELS

Here's a question for you: *How are you breathing?* Are you taking deep, even breaths, or do your breaths feel shallow? Checking in on your breathing is a helpful way to check in on your stress levels, so I invite you to pause and do this quick breathing activity.

Sitting upright, move your shoulders down and away from your ears. Take a deep breath in slowly through your nose. This breath should fill your belly, which is why sitting tall is helpful. If you find that your inhale is getting stuck in your chest, notice that. We'll come back to it. As you inhale deeply, imagine a balloon inflating in your midsection. When you've inhaled as much as you can without causing discomfort, use your mouth to exhale all that air, long and slow. Picture the balloon in your belly deflating as you breathe out.

Does that feel different from how you were breathing before? It does for me! Even as I type, I'm realizing that I haven't paused to take a deep breath in a while. I've been so focused on my work, hunched over my laptop, that my breaths have been short and shallow. Earlier today, while I was exercising, my breaths were shorter and faster to match my pace. When I recovered by stretching, my breaths shifted again, slower and deeper. Sometimes when I'm super stressed, it's hard for me to take a deep breath, and that's okay too. If you experienced that "stuck air" feeling in your chest when inhaling, your body might be giving you a hint about your stress levels.

Breathing is obviously essential to living, but what you may not realize is that the *way* you breathe is an indicator of how you're managing your stress. And you can use the way you breathe to intentionally shift your nervous system from a sympathetic (fight-flight-freeze-fawn) state to a parasympathetic (rest-and-digest) state. Learning how to manage my stress through breath work has been instrumental in my own healing journey, so I can't wait to share with you what I've learned! But first, let's talk about the purpose of breathing, because we must understand the *why* before we get to the *how*.

The Purpose of Breathing

The act of breathing is controlled by the autonomic nervous system, which means it's "automatic." Isn't it crazy that you don't have to remind your body to breathe? Your lungs expand and contract whether you tell them to or not. Because your breathing is connected to your nervous system, your state of stress impacts your breath rate and flow.

Think about it. When you get frustrated, you exhale loudly, pushing all your breath out in one burst. When you're focusing on something that involves intense concentration, your breath may become softer, with inhales and exhales shorter. When you engage in restful sleep (barring any sleep apnea), your breath rate changes to match the depth of your sleep.

Breathing is so instinctual that even the way our breath matches our state of stress feels natural. But before we get into how to use our breath to help manage our stress, it's important to understand the purpose of breathing—*why* and *how* we breathe—and how we can use it to help us heal.

Why We Breathe

At its most basic function, breathing is essential for keeping balance in the body. Breathing is how the body takes in oxygen for energy and expels carbon dioxide as part of its waste management system. Upon inhalation, air travels down the windpipe and into the bronchial tubes inside the lungs. When that happens, oxygen passes into the blood, and carbon dioxide is removed through exhalation. Every cell in your body uses oxygen to make energy, whereas excess carbon dioxide is a waste product that must be expelled to maintain homeostasis. Both oxygen and carbon dioxide are needed, but they must be in balance.

Well-oxygenated blood is more resistant to disease because it provides vital organs with better detoxification function. Deep breathing aids the lymphatic system in removing toxins from the body as well. Unlike the circulatory system, which functions automatically, the lymphatic system must be primed to function based on our movement and breathing practices. Because of our need to expel toxins through breath, breathing *out* is just as essential as breathing *in*.

In contrast to deep breathing, short and shallow mouth breathing limits oxygen intake to the upper lungs and reduces the efficiency of the gas exchange. Dr. Andrew Weil, a pioneer in integrative

Assess Your Breath

Need to breathe? Here are some indicators that you could benefit from mindful breath work. Check all that apply.

- ☐ I suffer from insomnia/wakefulness in the middle of the night.
- ☐ I struggle to fall asleep when I first go to bed.
- ☐ I rely on caffeine to keep me alert throughout the day.
- ☐ I wake up feeling exhausted, even when I sleep for eight hours or more.
- ☐ I have irregular bowel movements.
- ☐ I often feel distracted and unable to focus on a task.
- ☐ I can't seem to stick to a healthy eating plan because I always cave to cravings.
- ☐ I get unreasonably exhausted after I work out.
- ☐ I feel too exhausted to work out.
- ☐ I suffer from unstable blood sugar and bouts of hypoglycemia.
- ☐ The basic lab work at my annual exam changes from year to year and is trending in the wrong direction.
- ☐ I suffer from multiple food sensitivities or intolerances.
- ☐ I skip meals or eat too much.
- ☐ My menstrual cycle is irregular.
- ☐ My blood pressure is increasing.
- ☐ I am often anxious and concerned about perceived fears.
- ☐ I have bursts of energy some days, but other days I crash.

medicine, says, "If I had to limit my advice on healthier living to just one tip, it would be simply to learn how to breathe better."[1] In fact, breathing correctly matters so much that a two-decade study concluded, "The greatest indicator of life span wasn't genetics, diet, or the amount of daily exercise, as many had suspected. It was lung capacity."[2]

Why we breathe matters because without breath, we wouldn't have life; we wouldn't have internal balance. But *how* we breathe is what's most crucial for stress management and healing.

YOUR BREATH REFLECTS YOUR STRESS LEVELS

How We Breathe

Deep breathing is restorative. It can bring safety back to the body, especially after an acute stress exposure. Short, shallow breathing mimics a fight-or-flight state in the body, which is the natural response to threat, panic, or times when your brain is going faster than you can control. This kind of shallow breathing happens when your thoughts are bouncing around and varying from *What am I making for dinner?* to *That car better speed up or get out of my way!* to *I shouldn't have said that to her.*

Even the rate at which we breathe sends a message to the body about our state of stress. On average, we should be taking twelve breaths per minute, whereas overbreathing averages fifteen to eighteen breaths per minute.[3] Rapid overbreathing can throw off the oxygen-to-carbon-dioxide ratio and increase symptoms of anxiety or brain fog. It's another one of those brain-body, chicken-and-egg conundrums: Does stress cause breathing issues or do breathing issues cause more stress? I believe the answer is both. Even though breathing is automatic, we can hack into this process to work for us instead of against us.

Here's a quick stress check-in: As you're reading this, is your jaw clenched? Are your teeth clenched? If so, you'll have to intentionally unclench to take a deep breath. It's not possible to take long, slow, deep breaths through the nose when your teeth and jaw are clenched. It requires intentionality with the breath.

Here's another stress check-in: When you attempt a big inhale through your nose, do you feel that your breath gets stopped somewhere in your chest? Does it feel like there's a pressure or a weight there that you can't relieve? That's a signal that you're storing tension, and your body has become so accustomed to surviving with short, shallow breaths, it feels physically impossible to breathe any deeper. Your breath indicates survival mode.

Most of us (myself included) simply don't pause to check in

with ourselves—to notice our stress levels, to ask how we're feeling, and to assess our breathing patterns. We are conditioned to push through and keep going because the clock is ticking and there are things that must be done. We've got fancy paper calendars and planners, digital apps that tell us what's next, and notifications alerting us thirty minutes before our next scheduled appointment. With the handheld devices we carry everywhere, we get notified of world events as often as we want. There's no need for out-of-office email automations; we can work from our phones and respond to anything 24-7. Thanks to technology, we can multitask more efficiently than ever before. But while all that activity seems helpful on the surface, it simply perpetuates urgency and a sympathetic-dominant state in our brains and bodies.

Mindful breathing—focusing intentionally on your breathing—is something God designed to help your body get out of fight-or-flight mode and enter the parasympathetic state, rest-and-digest

The Vagus Nerve: A Gut-Brain Communication Highway

Vagus means "wandering" in Latin. The vagus nerve is the tenth cranial nerve that starts at the base of your skull and "wanders" all the way down to the gut. The wandering is purposeful, creating communication links between the brain and the digestive tract. That means that what happens in the vagus nerve doesn't stay in the vagus nerve. This nerve is responsive to the nervous system, creating a type of braking system for the sympathetic state (which triggers the fight-or-flight response) and helping the body calm the stress response. When you have high vagal tone (a higher capacity for stress), the vagus nerve responds to stress appropriately, activating the rest-and-digest state. When you have low vagal tone, the body is less stress resilient. Certain activities—singing, humming, gargling, and mindful breathing—can increase vagal tone.

mode. Breathing in through your nose, holding it, and exhaling through your mouth is the antidote to the fight-or-flight response in your body. It calms your vagus nerve—the nerve that runs from your brain all the way down to your gut and attaches to every organ along the way. Think of mindful breathing as an internal full-body massage that regulates your ability to handle stress.

Because the way that we breathe is automatic and changes with our stress levels, being mindful about our breath may feel strange at first—and, honestly, downright hard! We've all got at least ninety-nine problems to solve at any given time, and figuring out how to breathe through them isn't a task we want to add to our list. However, incorporating mindful breathing may be one of the most helpful things we can do to modulate the stress response throughout our day.

Take a Breath to Transition

One way to manage your stress is by using breath to transition from one activity to the next. Do busyness and a sense of hurry keep you from pausing to transition from one thing to the next during the day? Do you feel barraged by constant app notifications or interrupted by a stream of texts that constantly disrupt your focus? The myth of multitasking leads us to believe we are more efficient doing multiple things at once than we are doing one thing at a time. But what's the real outcome of multitasking? A dysregulated brain. Your brain can't fully concentrate on more than one thing. When you try to multitask, you grow scattered and unproductive, which brings anxiety and a lack of focus. Although the demands of contemporary life mean you will likely always have more than one plate spinning at a time and more than one task you need to complete in a given time frame, there are things you can do to regulate your brain and keep your focus.

Start making it a habit to pause and take a deep breath when you transition from one task to the next. When you're at home, going from kitchen to living room, pause and take a deep breath. When you're driving home and pull into your parking place or garage, pause and take a deep breath. When you're going from work to lunch, pause and take a deep breath. When you pause to breathe and make an active transition from one task to the other, you're more equipped to concentrate on the task at hand, which calms your nervous system and brings safety.

One example that daily reminds me of the importance of engaging in only one task at a time is chopping vegetables. Yes, the dreaded meal prep routine. I used to resent the time it took to cut vegetables for my meals because it felt like time I didn't have to spare. So I decided to take my own advice and try to make cutting veggies fun—a time to remain present in the moment. Sometimes I listen to a podcast or music, but mostly I chop in silence. I let my mind wander, and my breathing rate slows. It's a surprisingly effective mindfulness activity. I can only concentrate on one task, or I'll chop my finger off! Taking time to focus allows me to pay attention to the colors of the veggies, the smells, and the beauty in each different shape.

While concentrating on one task at a time is ideal, I'll be the first to acknowledge it's not always possible. For example, doing just one thing can be especially difficult as a parent. Every time I think I'm concentrating on just one thing, a child pops in to ask for food, help, permission to watch something, or to remind me they are bored. These interruptions can be frustrating, but it helps to think of them as simply another opportunity to practice breathing in transition.

Taking a moment to breathe as you transition from one task to the next can regulate your stress as you respond to alerts and interruptions throughout your day. If you go from one hurried activity to another without pausing and taking a deep breath, the overwhelm continues to build. Breathing to transition also helps to clear out the mental chatter by engaging the frontal lobe of the brain, which results in better decisions. Your nervous system equates deep and rhythmic breathing with safety, even on days when you feel like you're just doggy-paddling through. This is one quick way to partner with your body and brain and address your stress through breath.

Four Breathing Strategies to Address Stress

By now I hope you can see how pausing to breathe is the most accessible stress management tool you have. Breathing through your nose to flood your entire body with oxygen shifts your mental state, increasing awareness. But pausing to breathe during transitions is just one way to incorporate mindful breathing. There are also more focused breath work practices to explore.

Now comes the fun part! I'm going to give you some homework to try—four breathing exercises to help you check in with your stress daily. These are my go-to practices because they're easy to remember and can be used anytime.

The 4-7-8 breathing technique. This technique was made popular by Dr. Andrew Weil, and it was one of the first tools I learned in nutrition school. Find a comfortable seated position, legs uncrossed, hands open and resting on top of your thighs, spine straight. Inhale through your nose for four seconds, hold for seven seconds, and exhale through pursed lips for eight seconds. Do this for five rounds of inhales and exhales. Notice how your body responds after the first two rounds. Then notice how your body responds after the fifth round. Do you feel different? Less tense? This practice can also be done while lying down, especially if you're having a hard time going to sleep at night.

The physiological sigh. This natural pattern of breathing was identified by scientists in the 1930s but recently became popular due to the research of Dr. Andrew Huberman, a Stanford neuroscientist, who also is credited with naming it. This breathing method provides a way to shift our nervous system state when we're under stress. Inhale through your nose, and before you reach the top of the inhale, take another short inhale. Then do a long exhale through your mouth. I sometimes refer to this double-inhale style of breathing as a "cry sigh" because it's something we often do after a period of crying. It brings balance back to the nervous system naturally, and when you perform it intentionally while stressed, it can activate the parasympathetic (rest-and-digest) state in the body.

The bumblebee breath. This technique is specifically designed to support vagal tone by humming. A scientific study found it not only reduces stress but also reduces heart rate![4] Since practicing this one in public may make you feel a little conspicuous, save this for when you're alone. Sit up straight in a comfortable position and inhale through your nose. As you exhale, push your exhale out with a loud hum. Imagine that the humming sound sends vibrations all along the path of the vagus nerve, waking it up and activating the parasympathetic nervous system state. I find that doing just three rounds of this is soothing.

Alternate nostril breathing. While sitting in a comfortable position, legs uncrossed, bring your right hand up to your nose. Place your thumb on your right nostril, blocking it from receiving air. Inhale deeply, sending all the air into your left nostril. Then, as you hold the inhale, release your thumb from your right nostril and use your middle finger to block your left nostril; exhale through the right nostril. Next, repeat the process in reverse. Block the left nostril with your middle finger as you inhale through the right nostril. On the exhale, block the right nostril with your thumb and exhale through the left. Continue that cycle for as many rounds as you need. One scientific study found that this exercise not only increases relaxation but also brings focus and alertness![5] This may be a great exercise to use when you need some extra calm while concentrating on a big project or task.

Your body is so kind to send you red flags through mental and physical symptoms. Intentional breathing is a way to respond back to the body, letting it know you saw the flag and you're in this together. Whatever physical or mental health condition you may be struggling with, using breath to shift your mental state can be a helpful tool in your healing journey. Remember, breath equals safety; and slow, deep breathing reminds your body you don't have to be in survival mode.

MAKING THE MIND-BODY CONNECTION

Choose one of the four breathing exercises to focus on for one day—the 4-7-8 breathing technique, the physiological sigh, the bumblebee breath, or alternate nostril breathing. Set a reminder on your phone to stop and use your breathing exercise at regular intervals throughout the day. For example, when you wake up, midmorning, lunchtime, midafternoon, dinnertime, and before bed. If you forget or miss one, don't beat yourself up. Remember to keep a mindset of observation and curiosity, not self-criticism. Evaluate how taking regular breathing breaks impacts you—your experience of stress, ability to focus, sense of well-being, and so on.

PART 2

LEARN to address stress

IDENTIFY THE ROOT ISSUES

add VARIETY to your diet

EXERCISE your body and brain

Have you ever seen an illustration of an iceberg? The portion of the iceberg that is visible above the water is only about 10 percent of the total mass, which doesn't even come close to accurately portraying the iceberg's true depth and width under the water. Hence, the cliché, "It's just the tip of the iceberg." When it comes to your labels, naming them is truly just the tip of the iceberg. Your labels have many under-the-surface factors driving their presentation—and those factors, the root issues, could be the reasons you get stuck and feel held back in your healing.

In part 2, we're diving deep. But I'm not going to take you anywhere I haven't journeyed myself. We're in this together. We'll start with the stories and core beliefs you've developed to cope with any trauma you may have experienced. We'll tackle your coping mechanisms and why you can't seem to change the things you want to change. And we'll explore how to reacquaint yourself with blocked feelings and what to do when all the promised magic fixes fail.

Be sure to make time to practice the mind-body exercises included at the end of each chapter. While they're not magic fixes, they will keep you connected with your body and grounded in truth as you dig deep to break through the layers of *why*.

Now, let's get the diving gear out and take the plunge under the surface. I think you may discover some things you haven't considered before.

6

IS IT ME OR MY TRAUMA RESPONSE?

When I was four years old, my family went on a road trip in our Toyota station wagon. We lived in central California at the time, and we drove south to visit Disneyland and my grandparents in Orange County. My parents loaded the luggage on top of the car and strapped it down. They buckled up me, and my two-year-old twin sister and brother, and we experienced a magical trip. Unfortunately, on the way home the luggage became dislodged and flew all over the highway. Our clothes, souvenirs, and the ring my grandma had given my mom as a high school graduation gift were lost.

    Strangely enough, I don't remember that part. But here's what I do remember: We stopped at a gas station soon after, and my parents asked me to wait in the car with my siblings while they went inside to make a phone call. With my anxious, overthinking, hyperalert, and self-protective brain, I could tolerate sitting there for probably fifteen seconds. Then, fearful that someone would kidnap me (even though my parents likely had me in their vision the whole time), I rushed inside to find them. It was only when I came back out that I realized the luggage on top of the car was gone. In my four-year-old mind, I believed the luggage had vanished because I left the car, which allowed some bad guys to steal it. For probably a decade, I believed that the lost luggage was my fault—that my tiny self would have been a deterrent to luggage thieves, which was why my parents had asked me to wait in the car.

I believed the wrong story for a long time. I believed a self-invented lie because I needed to make sense of the world around me. I didn't understand my parents' panic and anxiety, so I made it my fault.

Editing our stories to understand them better is a very human behavior, especially for anyone who has experienced trauma. We edit and recreate stories from major life experiences so we have an understandable category in which to file them away. It's a helpful survival response, but it's not always as simple as a child making sense of lost luggage.

Here's another example, and this one is a little more complicated: For many years, I shut out memories of sexual assault that happened to me in early adulthood when my mental state was at its lowest point. To make sense of the chaos, I painted myself as the villain. I blamed myself and took ownership for what happened, even though I was the victim and easy prey because of unfortunate circumstances, my deteriorating mental state, prescription medications, and alcohol abuse. Due to early life trauma, I used a common trauma coping mechanism, dissociation, to check out—which means I separated my brain from my body for self-protection. This made it more difficult to recall events accurately. When the memories did eventually reemerge, I experienced them as if I were watching a video of someone else. It felt surreal and hard to believe. But once again, I made it my fault.

Many people who struggle with mood disorders, manic episodes, and substance abuse also struggle with reality—with distinguishing the facts of what happened from their memories of what happened. Memories can be unreliable, especially when medications and other substances are involved. Looking for a narrative that makes sense can feel like dodging cars on a busy highway in search of a lost piece of jewelry—both dangerous and futile. Trauma—and the dissociation we often use to cope with it—alters the narrative and creates a new but distorted story to make sense of the most unimaginable situations.

The impact of trauma doesn't just affect how we view our stories; it impacts the response of our nervous systems. This often creates dysregulation that begs the question, Is it me or my trauma response?

Living in a Trauma Response

While everyone will experience trauma at some point in their lives, not everyone will experience *symptoms* of post-traumatic stress disorder (PTSD) or get the diagnostic *label* of PTSD.[1] But know this: Even without an official diagnosis of PTSD, we can still live in a perpetual trauma response. A trauma response is your nervous system's adaptation to a traumatic event. As you recall, an immediate response to a threat is the sympathetic activation of the fight-flight-freeze-fawn state; and after the threat has passed, the body can enter back into a parasympathetic state.

Unfortunately, because of how trauma is imprinted into the nervous system, we can lose nervous system flexibility and the ability to move from sympathetic back to parasympathetic. Because traumatic experiences are stored in our nervous system to protect against future threats—and we know the brain and body are always communicating—we need to understand the impact of trauma on both our physical and emotional well-being.

The Impact of Trauma on Emotional Well-Being

The emotional impact of trauma is far-reaching and looks different for each person affected by it. Because of this, many clinicians attempt to differentiate between what is sometimes referred to as "big T" trauma and "little t" trauma. Big T trauma refers to experiencing major events, such as war, witnessing murder or death, rape, robbery, recurring abuse, racism, or natural disasters. Little t trauma refers to experiences such as rejection, bullying, harsh parenting, medical issues, embarrassment, or moving.

I'm not a fan of distinguishing between big T trauma and little t trauma because no matter the event or the cause, it's the *impact* of the event that determines whether there's a feeling of safety or feelings associated with hypervigilance. The individual's *felt response*, rather than the event itself, is what matters. That's why two people who experience the same event might have very different responses—one traumatic and the other not.

The emotional impact on those who experience trauma might range from being easily shut down or overly activated. For some, emotions might feel completely blocked or easily bruised. Others may feel more easily overwhelmed or have a strong need to power through no matter what they're feeling. Trauma can also diminish emotional capacity, making it much more difficult to stay regulated when faced with perceived threats that "bump against" a traumatic memory. There's a physiological reason for that: The brain stores traumatic memories differently.

New research shows that traumatic memories are stored in the brain differently than memories that are merely sad. The hippocampus is the part of the brain that stores memory, and the amygdala tags the memory with sensory details, such as smell, sound, taste, touch, or sight. That's why smelling a specific scent or hearing a familiar song on the radio might quickly pull up a memory associated with that scent or song. When it comes to trauma, though, reexperiencing the memory activates a different part of the brain, the posterior cingulate cortex (PCC).

The PCC is involved in narrative comprehension, autobiographical processing, and emotional memory imagery. In other words, the PCC plays a role in how you make sense of your story, especially the parts of your story that are more emotionally charged, such as traumatic memories. According to one researcher, "The brain does not treat traumatic memories as regular memories, or perhaps even as memories at all."[2] For someone suffering from trauma, a traumatic flashback can feel like it's happening in real time. Because the brain didn't process the memory according to its typical memory filing system, its ability to comprehend the narrative and process the events in a linear fashion is altered.

This means traumatic memories have a heavier emotional impact than regular memories. Because such memories can feel like ever-present warning alerts, emotional regulation can be more difficult, resulting in more frequent mood changes, hypervigilance, anxiety, and distractibility. Diagnostic labels such as major depressive disorder, generalized anxiety disorder, bipolar disorder, schizophrenia, and others can be a result of trauma's emotional toll. While the brain is fighting off potential triggers and defending itself with hypervigilance, it takes up a lot of emotional bandwidth, which becomes draining. Perhaps two of the most draining impacts of trauma on emotional well-being are hypersensitivity and shame.

Trauma can set you up for hypersensitivity to other people's emotions.[3] The impact is twofold: While trauma can cause you to be even more highly sensitive and empathetic to others' pain, the increased sensitivity can also lead to a more difficult time processing and recovering from anything that triggers emotional intensity. If you've ever been told, "You're being too sensitive," you know it can feel like an insult to your identity. You didn't choose your highly sensitive responses. You're not faking your sensitivity. It is a learned response that keeps you alerted to danger in order to protect you from it.

Another emotional side effect of trauma is shame. Shame, in the context of trauma, is the internalization that because something bad happened to you, *you* are bad. Shame rewrites your story so that you believe that you are beyond healing, beyond love, and beyond all hope for repair. Shame also prevents you from being vulnerable in your relationships, especially your relationship with your heavenly Father. Shame can even prevent you from seeing the truth about your identity—that you are a child of God—and living in that truth. Shame will stunt any growth or progress you make, because when you take a step forward, shame is lurking in the back of your mind, telling you exactly why you can't and won't succeed. Shame reminds you that you're the broken one. And yet, as crazy as it sounds, shame is a protective response, because focusing all the attention on you as the problem or villain allows you to avoid dealing with the deeper hurt you experienced.

I witnessed the emotional impact of trauma-based shame in my client Laura. For years, she struggled with a need to control her environment to feel good about herself. She worked to check every box with her health and didn't understand why she still struggled with hormonal imbalances. She ate the "right things" and exercised daily. But after she shared her story with me, I learned that a trauma to her body early in life caused her to internalize the message that her body was bad. Her shame about her body led her to do everything she could to control it. Her emotional stress created a physiological stress response in her body that impacted her hormones. Her symptoms eventually improved, but her healing required that she treat herself more gently. She needed to address the shame, and at the root of the shame was the trauma response.

The Impact of Trauma on Physical Well-Being

The experiences and corresponding emotional pain your body holds impact so much more than your brain. *Neuroception*, a term coined by Dr. Stephen Porges, refers to the process by which the nervous system subconsciously scans for signs of safety or danger. Trauma alters neuroception by creating a deep, felt sense of unsafety at the physical level—even when we have no logical reason to feel unsafe. And once again, this demonstrates another aspect of our protective design.

Here's a personal example of how trauma impacts neuroception. While most people enjoy the beauty and scent of honeysuckles, I spent many years trying to avoid them. Smelling the fresh bloom of honeysuckles every spring instantly took me back to the day I was nine and stood frozen at my front window watching my grandpa die of anaphylaxis and wondering when God would show up to save him. As a protective measure, my neuroception had been altered by the trauma of my grandpa's death so that my body now associated the scent of honeysuckles with danger. Thanks to the trauma therapy Eye Movement Desensitization and Reprocessing (EMDR), that memory has been refiled in my brain.[4] It's still a sad memory, but the sight and smell of honeysuckles no longer trigger the same overwhelming freeze response.

Your body remembers what your brain struggles to process and categorize. Your body can feel signals of danger, even when you're doing everything you can mentally to heal. I've lost count of the number of clients who've told me something like, "I've been to talk therapy. I've processed my trauma. I'm saying all the positive things and working on my self-talk. So why does it seem like my body doesn't feel safe? Why does it feel like my body is working against me?" On the surface, they're doing all the things they're supposed to be doing, but they struggle to feel calm or settled because their body feels restless and charged, alert for any sign of danger.

Another example of the physical impact of trauma comes from the delayed impact of adverse childhood experiences. The Adverse Childhood Experiences (ACE) study showed that events such as abuse, neglect, and dysfunction that happen in childhood may predispose a person to negative health outcomes later in life. In 2019, the Centers for Disease Control and Prevention (CDC) found that at least five of the top ten leading causes of death, including respiratory and heart disease, cancer, and suicide, are associated with adverse childhood experiences.[5]

Remember in chapter 3 when we talked about the gut-brain axis and psychoneuroimmunology? Trauma disrupts the microbial balance in the gut, leading to enhanced intestinal permeability. This creates physiological stress in the GI tract and interferes with gut-brain signaling. It can even increase risk of autoimmune disease due to the way it creates a hypervigilant alert in the immune system. As Dr. Sara Gottfried writes, "Your body stores the trauma in your brain, stress response, hormonal control system, immune system, and nervous system."[6]

Lifetime priming of the amygdala (the emotional response and reaction portion of the brain) happens in childhood and even informs baseline metabolism. This means your current cellular communication and energy expenditure can highly depend on the information you received about the world as a child. If your brain determined that you were unsafe, your amygdala was primed to let your body know—from metabolic function to digestive health to reproductive hormones and even immune system health. Stored trauma shows up even in your DNA.[7] For example, one study showed that PTSD can change the expression of genes, altering stress response and the immune system.[8]

When it comes to trauma, there is a whole-body symphony showing up to keep you alerted to danger—anytime, anywhere. Another consequence of these chronic alerts is the compartmentalization of emotional and physical symptoms, which I refer to as the emotional-physical split.

The Emotional-Physical Split

The mind-body connection can be ruptured because of trauma. This makes so much sense. If your body isn't a safe place, why would your mind choose to be in it? If your body is constantly in a survival state, on high alert to respond to emotional and physical triggers that remind your brain and body of past traumatic experiences, then compartmentalization can occur.

Compartmentalization is a defense mechanism we choose (consciously or subconsciously) to separate our body and mind from conflicting emotions, physical discomfort, and experiences that cause distress. This compartmentalization can lead to living in an "autopilot" state, disconnected from the body and its needs. For example, many of us trauma survivors hate sitting down or being still because too much inactivity or silence makes those zaps of unsafety too loud. So we stay busy. This allows us to create and maintain a disconnect between body and brain.

Another way to compartmentalize is through dissociation, which is what I did to avoid being present in my body during early life medical trauma. Dissociation disconnects you from thoughts, feelings, memories, and even your identity. When life gets overwhelming, you check out. You may feel like you're watching yourself from outside your body. You might isolate or limit contact with loved ones for a time. Dissociation is protective, because bad things don't happen to you if you're not completely there.

I didn't know I had patterns of dissociation until my thirties. For most of my life, I just thought I was spacey. When I was growing up, my family and friends had a name for my dissociative stare. They called it "The Zone." When it happened, I would hear people talking about me, saying things like, "Guys, she's in The Zone again." The person who said it would be right in front of me, but I heard them from far away, as if on the other side of a long tunnel. I never did it on purpose, and I never knew what triggered it. My friend Amanda took a picture of me at a party during our senior year of high school, where I'm clearly in the middle of a game of pool, yet I'm standing still, staring blankly ahead, deep in The Zone. I had no memory of zoning out until the picture was later developed and Amanda gave it to me.

When your body doesn't feel safe, living with a fully integrated mind, body, and spirit is scary. Being present in your body feels foreign. Compartmentalization and dissociation are coping mechanisms that help you to feel safe.

Living in a perpetual trauma response impacts many of your emotional and physical symptoms. But before you can facilitate the healing process and move forward, you must make room to grieve the loss of a trauma-free life.

Make Space for Grief

The good news is that just as trauma rewires the brain and body, so can healing. Because so many of us want to press fast-forward on our healing, we often miss an important step. That step is experiencing grief. The American Psychological Association defines grief as "the anguish experienced after significant loss, usually the death of a beloved person. . . . Grief may also take the form of regret for something lost, remorse for something done, or sorrow for a mishap to oneself."[9]

With trauma comes loss. Loss of *what* could have been and loss of who *you* could have been. There are stories you will never have because of the stories you were forced to live. It is a courageous act of self-compassion to make space to grieve the losses you experienced in the wake of trauma.

If you're like me and many of my clients who are trauma survivors, you may not have allowed yourself that space to grieve. It's much more common to push through and minimize the trauma, saying things like, "It could've been worse. I survived, and I'm fine." Or, "It's not as bad as what's happening on the other side of the world." Or to use clichés such as, "What doesn't kill you makes you stronger" or, "God gives his toughest battles to his strongest warriors."

Suppressing emotional pain and minimizing trauma might make you feel safe mentally, but tending to your nervous system to restore whole-body safety requires acknowledging and experiencing grief. Unlike the act of grieving after the loss of a person, a season, or even a job, you may need to grieve *yourself*. Traumatic experiences can completely alter your view of yourself and how you experience safety in your body. These experiences can shift your story and rewrite your core beliefs, which often creates additional negative labels.

Instead of choosing avoidance and compartmentalization, you may need to grieve your old story to find safety from the constant trigger alerts and to walk into a new story. This means acknowledging how your pain and your core beliefs merge to shape the way the story plays out.

If you believe you are a bother, due to your emotional needs being unmet as a child, you might struggle to reach out to others for help. This belief will keep you in a state of self-sufficiency with a need for control. But before you can edit the story to find healing, you may need to pause and grieve for the child who didn't get her emotional needs met.

You might believe that you are too much, because you've suffered from endless medical issues for many years, living at the mercy of appointments, prescriptions, and attempted solutions. Before you can edit the story that you are too much, maybe you need to grieve the loss of health in your life. You may need to grieve the loss of hopes and dreams of healing. You may need to grieve for what could have been.

Perhaps you believe the story that you are unlovable, because you didn't receive love in the way you needed it—you received a skewed and conditional version of it, or you received love based on

What It Means to Grieve Your Story

Grieving your story requires acknowledging the loss that trauma caused. There are five stages of grief: denial, bargaining, anger, depression, and acceptance. The order in which we experience those stages differs from person to person and from one experience to the next. Here are what the five stages look like through the lens of trauma:

Denial: "That didn't happen to me. I'm fine. I don't have trauma. My childhood wasn't that bad, not like some people's."

Bargaining: "If only I hadn't said yes to going to that party. If only I hadn't gone to school that day. If only I hadn't been born to that family."

Anger: "Why didn't they see how hurt I was? How could they do that to me? I'm so frustrated with myself for letting that happen."

Depression: "I don't know if I'll ever make it past this."

Acceptance: "I went through a really tough time. I'm sad that it happened, but I can also learn to comfort myself moving forward and recognize when I'm feeling triggered."

Ultimately, acceptance is where we want to land, but we might bounce around in some of the other stages before we get there. It is okay to experience the different stages of grief as you look back at your story and acknowledge the role trauma played in it. Let yourself process those feelings by journaling, talking through your experiences with a trusted friend, or making an appointment with a licensed counselor.

achievement or merit. This may keep you from actively engaging in safe, healthy relationships. Before you can heal, you may need to grieve for the person who never got to know what unconditional love really means.

It's possible that you've never felt you had permission to grieve—especially if your trauma happened in childhood. Acknowledging the loss is a compassionate way to create room for a new story. It creates room to support your nervous system's felt sense of safety as a pathway to healing.

Understanding the impact of trauma on your nervous system is an important step to addressing the root issues that hold you back from making progress in your healing journey. Trauma's imprint is another threat alerting your brain to danger and signaling unrest in your body. Whether you're experiencing emotional or physical symptoms of the trauma response, I hope acknowledging trauma as one root cause will help you view your story with both self-compassion and hope moving forward.

MAKING THE MIND-BODY CONNECTION

Releasing stored trauma requires a whole-body approach. While your body doesn't know the difference between a real or perceived threat, it also doesn't know the difference between a current threat or the threat of a traumatic memory that has been imprinted in your mind. Your body won't feel safe until it experiences regular and intentional safety.

What follows is a mind-body technique to help your body and brain process truth statements based on God's Word, which is "alive and active" (Hebrews 4:12, NIV). If unprocessed trauma is a root issue for you, I encourage you to find a therapist who is trained in trauma, specifically in somatic healing. EMDR and Emotional Freedom Technique (EFT), or tapping, are two of the most well-known, evidence-based tools to support healing from trauma. However, there are also newer somatic processing techniques, such as Somatic Experiencing, and some researchers have found promising results in the use of psychedelics to help lessen the effect of trauma.

The technique I'd like you to try is called "butterfly taps." It's designed to engage bilateral stimulation (alternately activating both sides of your brain) with gentle tapping as you reframe one of your labels.

Listed below are a series of paired statements, each one representing a core belief often associated with trauma, and a truth from Scripture that counters that core belief. As you read through the statements, pay attention to both your mind and your body. Circle one or two of the statements that resonate most with you.

Core Belief from Trauma	Truth from Scripture
I am alone.	I am safe with my Father (Romans 8:15).
I am helpless.	I am protected (Psalm 27:5).
I am unworthy.	I am made worthy by Jesus' power (2 Corinthians 12:9).
I am unlovable.	I am loved and known (1 John 4:16).
I am not enough.	I am more than a conqueror (Romans 8:1, 37).
I am too much.	I am filled with the Spirit (2 Corinthians 1:21-22).
I am beyond healing.	I am being made new every day (2 Corinthians 4:16).
I am broken.	I am his workmanship (Ephesians 2:10).
I am damaged goods.	I am restored (Romans 6:4).
I am a bother.	I am welcome to approach the throne (Hebrews 4:16).
I am a lost cause.	I am redeemed (2 Corinthians 5:17).
I am a victim.	I am rescued (Psalm 91:14-15).
I am a villain.	I am a friend of God (John 15:15).

IS IT ME OR MY TRAUMA RESPONSE?

Choose one of the statements you circled to focus on and process it with butterfly taps as follows:

- Take a deep breath in through your nose and let it out through your mouth.
- Cross your hands over your chest so that the tips of your fingers rest just beneath your collarbones.
- As you say the core belief statement out loud, begin to tap with your fingertips, alternating taps on your left and right sides, just beneath your collarbones. Then say the truth out loud, as you continue to tap right, left, right, left, as many times as you need to.
- Take another deep breath in through your nose and let it out through your mouth.
- Check in with yourself and notice any thoughts and feelings.

Use this practice as often as needed as a reminder of the truth of your identity.

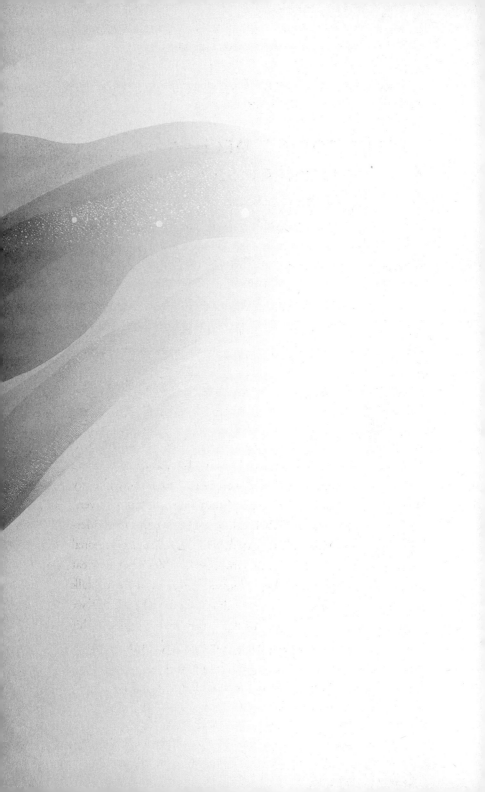

7
THE COPING MECHANISMS THAT KEPT YOU SAFE

"I'm pretty sure I have a food addiction," said my new client, Ben, describing his daily food intake. I always ask about daily eating habits the first time I meet with someone. People seek out my help for a variety of health issues, and looking at their food inventory gives me a snapshot of their eating habits. It helps me understand likes and dislikes, daily patterns, and the client's emotional relationship with food. The way someone describes what they eat can also clue me in to lifestyle patterns and even negative self-talk that may be roadblocks on their healing journey when and if we begin to discuss diet changes. In Ben's case, he felt stalled in his health and believed his food habits were the culprit. I suspected that there was a lot more going on than overdoing it on certain foods. I wanted to dig deeper to the root of why he felt like he was getting tripped up by food.

"What makes you think you have a food addiction?" I asked.

"I don't know when to stop," he said. "I don't think I even eat when I'm hungry. I just pick things because they taste good, and then I eat them without really thinking about whether they're good for me or not."

I nodded and smiled in recognition. It wasn't the first time I'd heard this type of comment. "What do you think is behind that?"

He shrugged. "I really don't know. I guess it's just an addiction problem."

Like Ben, many of my clients struggle with knowing what they're supposed to eat and how to control what they eat. Overconsumption of food for comfort is one type of habit that is deeply personal and often rooted in childhood habits and beliefs. I completely understand the struggle because I, too, have experienced what it's like to feel out of control with what I considered to be bad habits.

As a teenager, I spent long hours hidden away from the world with books—to the extent that I turned down invitations to parties my senior year of high school to get lost in a world of fiction. Like Ben, I thought I had a discipline problem or just bad habits. I berated myself for the things I did that I didn't want to do, and I longed to be able to make consistent changes. It took me years to realize that there were other factors at play in my body and brain. Looking back, I would say that I didn't have bad habits so much as I had a lot of coping mechanisms that kept me safe when my nervous system was overwhelmed. However, these coping mechanisms led me to chronic self-bullying. It wasn't until I learned to reframe the way I thought about my "bad habits" that everything fell into place.

Getting to the Root of Bad Habits

To get to the root of your health issues—before making drastic changes—it's helpful to evaluate why you do what you do (in a gentle, self-compassionate way, of course). Maybe you, like many people I work with, want to make changes to feel better, but you get tripped up by behavioral patterns that halt your progress. These behaviors are likely coping mechanisms, and they serve a purpose.

Coping mechanisms are behaviors we develop to manage stress. They are the routines, rituals, or habits we accumulate over time to make our days more manageable. Because everyone's capacity for stress is different, the patterned behaviors we use to cope with our stress are different too. Some people rely on coffee in the morning to get going while others might go for a run or make a to-do list for the day. Some people enjoy a sweet treat after a long day and others take a hot bath. None of these attempts to manage stress are bad. However, when our coping mechanisms start to interfere with our functioning, they can turn into what we call our bad habits. And those habits keep us stuck. What I've discovered in working with my clients over the years is that bad habits don't just pop up out of nowhere. They arise primarily from two things: a deep need for comfort and a faulty core belief system.

Bad Habits Indicate a Need for Comfort

What if I told you that your bad habit, the one you want to change, is not a bad habit—that it is instead an old friend? And your old friend has brought you comfort through various seasons of life. Would this change how you think about it? Let me share a few stories that demonstrate what I mean.

Monica is a mom of three young children who feels addicted to her afternoon trip to the coffee shop drive-through. The baristas expect her and know her order. When she made an appointment with me, she was struggling with anxiety and an inability to get restful sleep. She thought she had a caffeine problem that made things worse. What we uncovered about her caffeine habit was that she wanted a treat—one that was hers alone and that she didn't have to share. The habit started not long after the birth of her first child and had become a ritual she looked forward to, especially on long days of handling toddler meltdowns and diaper changes. The "old friend" brought her comfort. Cutting out her ritual might decrease her evening anxiety and sleep problems, but understanding her need for comfort helped her to make changes in a way that stuck.

Sasha is a recently divorced woman in her fifties whose habit involves winding down with Netflix and falling asleep to one of her favorite comedy series. She explained it was the only way she could get to sleep, because she didn't like the silence of her house at night. She wanted to improve her bedtime routine to feel more rested in the morning. Her lab results also revealed high cortisol levels, which indicated a need for stress management. However, before drastically changing her habit, we did some digging. We discovered that falling asleep to the TV is an old friend. As a child, she often went to sleep in front of the TV to drown out the sounds of her parents fighting in the other room. The TV helped her to feel like she wasn't alone.

Elizabeth, a thirty-year-old fifth-grade teacher, is feeling burned out by the demands of her job. When she gets home from teaching, overstimulated and exhausted, she takes a nap that often lasts past dinnertime. As a result, she ends up with little time or energy for cooking and meal prepping for her workdays. So she relies on nutrient-poor convenience foods, which leave her feeling even more exhausted—and the cycle perpetuates. Before we could discuss strategies to make her life more manageable, we needed to discuss her old friends. The convenience foods she gravitates toward most turned out to be foods that reminded her of her childhood, when life was simpler and less stressful. At the root of her habits is a need for comfort.

My oldest coping strategy friend comes in the form of a good book and a snack. In high school, when my moods were

THE COPING MECHANISMS THAT KEPT YOU SAFE

unpredictable and I longed to fall into a deep dark hole and not come out until the world looked happy again, I took a lot of "off days." Depression showed up in mystery sickness, though I discovered many years later that it's not a mystery when you understand the physical symptoms of trauma and even the inflammatory nature of depression or anxiety. At one point during my senior year of high school, I was absent one day each week. My friends wrote "Erin's Off Day" on a card and set it at my empty desk. On the back of the card, they wrote all the various reasons I gave for being absent. I'm pretty sure one of them was, "I need to take a big poop," though I for sure never said that was why I was staying home. When life got overwhelming, I shut down and hid out. My books and snacks of pretzel mixes and sour candy filled a void for me. Through them, I got out of my head and into a safe place. This became a way for me to isolate and shut other people out, which is a habit that followed me into adulthood—even into my marriage.

My guess is that you, like so many of us, have some habits you'd like to change. You may even consider them a hindrance on your health journey and therefore feel ashamed by your inability to overcome them. Perhaps your habits are the focus of your negative self-talk, or enemies you feel like you need to defeat before your life can be better, healthier, and whole. However you think of them, would you be willing, even if just for a moment, to view these coping mechanisms as your old friends? Because as crazy as it may sound, you likely *needed* your bad habits for a season of your life.

I am grateful for the comfort I once received from my old friends. As an adolescent, I spent so much of my energy trying to achieve, to appear competent, and to control outcomes that the relief I felt when I shut down with a book and some food kept me from going into a much more dangerous place during depressive states. Unfortunately, shutting down and avoiding people isn't a solid strategy for adulting—not to mention marriage and parenting hardships.

My guess is that your bad habits aren't new—that they, or some version of them, have been sources of comfort, escape, or companionship for a very long time. Your coping mechanisms may have filled a void during a time you felt depleted, afraid, or lonely. They may have offered you support when you felt little support, or perhaps they were tools you used to manage big emotions you didn't know what to do with. It's okay to have coping mechanisms; the problem comes when the behaviors start to bring more consequences than comfort, more dysfunction than peace. When old friends become needy friends that keep you stuck, it may be that you have outgrown them, and it's time to let them go.

Take a moment and consider:

- How have your coping mechanisms been a friend to you? How have they served you or brought you comfort during a time when you needed it?

- In what ways do your coping mechanisms no longer serve you? Or in what ways might you have outgrown them? Consider any ways in which they contribute to you feeling stuck or unable to live the life you want.

- What thoughts or emotions come to mind when you imagine yourself saying goodbye to your old friends?

When you can imagine your coping mechanisms as old friends who no longer fit into this season of growth and change, it helps reframe things in a gentler way. When you view your habits as old friends rather than enemies, you can offer yourself compassion and care and explore the purpose these old friends played in your life. When you can reframe your bad habits as old friends who no longer serve you, you can say goodbye and move forward into new habits.

Bad Habits Connect to Faulty Core Beliefs

Coping mechanisms are often connected to faulty core beliefs, especially those that arise because of trauma or other negative experiences. Remember, core beliefs are deeply held and often rigid beliefs about ourselves and the world around us. They can become so entrenched in the brain that they impact our behaviors and how we choose to cope with the world, especially when we're overwhelmed by emotional and physiological stress. And when our core beliefs are faulty, they can create a vicious cycle of coping from deficiency.

For example, if your faulty core belief is that you are not enough, your resulting coping mechanism might show up as overconfidence and perfectionism. You feel driven to accomplish and achieve, and your nonstop pace of life demonstrates that. Your behaviors may give others the impression that you are capable and efficient, but the imposter syndrome you experience only perpetuates your belief that you're not enough. What started out as a need for efficiency now becomes the coping mechanism of trying to appear so overly efficient that it becomes a chronic stressor.

If your faulty core belief is that you are unworthy or unloved, your coping mechanism might look like going out of your way to help, even at the expense of caring for your own needs. As a result, you're often left feeling completely drained, which only drives you to look for more service opportunities to help you feel better again. What appears to be a helpful coping mechanism on the surface can end up creating internal chaos.

If your faulty core belief is that you are unseen, then your coping mechanism might drive you to do what you can to be noticed, get the accolades, and find success. But once the spotlight fades, you still feel unseen and must strive for more recognition and success. Once again, a protective coping mechanism leads to inner dissatisfaction.

Sometimes being caught up in negative core beliefs can lead to inactivity and shutdown, especially when all your efforts to compensate for your deficiency go unnoticed or appear to be wasted. For example, if your faulty core belief is that you are "less than" or not enough, and your life experiences continue to reaffirm that message to you over time, you may feel completely immobilized and trapped. Or you may go through life in survival mode, doing just the bare minimum to stay afloat. This may lead to relying on mood-altering substances (such as caffeine, overly processed foods, alcohol, prescription medication, and recreational drugs) just to make it through the disappointment you experience.

Your core beliefs drive your current habits and cognitions, whether positive or negative. They keep you in a familiar pattern of being, one that feels safe, because your life experiences affirm the faulty belief you have about yourself. Unfortunately, such core beliefs can keep you from living authentically—as the person God created you to be—because you're functioning out of a deficit. When your worth constantly feels threatened, you feel the need to wear a mask to show up for daily duties. In addition to depleting your limited energy by constantly trying to compensate for a deficit, the lack of authenticity prevents you from being truly yourself with others—which means you're cut off from a source of primary nourishment.

Getting rid of bad habits isn't as simple as eliminating the behavior holding you back. When you dig into the root cause of the habit, whether it's a need for comfort or a negative core belief, what you discover can help you to identify the specific unmet need that fuels your struggle. It allows you to partner with your body and brain to make changes that stick. But it isn't easy. Making changes requires a complex yet fascinating process that occurs in your brain, using the neurotransmitter dopamine.

Why Training Your Brain to Change Is So Hard

Perhaps you're thinking, "Hey, Erin. Getting to the root of my issues sounds cool and everything, but for real: How do I stop craving sugar? Why can't I say no?"

Well, I'm so glad you asked because we've come to my favorite part: addressing how we can train the brain to change. There's a reason we get hooked on coping mechanisms, and it all starts with one of my favorite neurotransmitters: dopamine. Dopamine is a neurotransmitter that affects motivation, pleasure, and how we get things done. When we understand this aspect of the brain's reward system and partner with the other root causes of our habits, it can help us put all the pieces together to make change happen. *For real.*

Research shows that dopamine simultaneously affects both learning and motivation.[1] And this makes sense because if we had no chemical messenger modulating our motivation, we would have no reason to work and get things done. Because dopamine is connected to our reward centers, when we experience pleasure from a reward, our brains want to do that thing again so we can experience the same feeling of pleasure.

This is the reward system that brought my client Monica comfort from her afternoon iced latte. It's why my client Elizabeth reverted to her favorite childhood foods when she felt overwhelmed. Their brains knew that those behaviors would reward them with comfort. And the same dynamic is true for you and me. Caving to a hit of dopamine when we feel depleted is what sabotages the new habits we want to implement.

Dopamine signaling—a process in which the neurotransmitter dopamine transmits signals between neurons in the brain—happens both in anticipation of doing something that brings pleasure as well as in the act of doing the thing. A perfect example of this is food. We're motivated to make our favorite meal because we know we'll enjoy it; hence, the phrase "comfort food." Then when we eat that meal, it triggers a feeling of pleasure in the brain, and the brain stores that memory and asks for more later to repeat the feeling.

The challenge we face that generations before us haven't is that some of our favorite foods have been engineered to be richer and sweeter than anything found in nature, so they *overstimulate* the reward system and "hook us" to go back for more—and in ever-increasing amounts. This same overstimulation dynamic has also proven true for other modern realities such as social media and streaming entertainment. That's why we can't stop scrolling and end up deciding to watch "just one more episode." We keep pushing for that hit of dopamine, always craving more, while eventually feeling completely out of control, like we're sabotaging anything we want to change. *Too much of a good thing can truly be too much.*

Some of us tend to be more affected by dopamine signaling than others, so we run through the effects of the stimulation more rapidly, leading to a greater need for "new and shiny" objects. We get bored easily, or we don't like sitting still, or life frequently feels overwhelming, so we turn to those quick hits to keep us moving forward. In terms of human development, this is an effective survival strategy, but over time it can lead to discouragement and disappointment when we just can't seem to quit the thing we want to quit.

The more dysregulated your nervous system is, the more you long for that dopamine hit. This creates a type of seeking-getting-seeking cycle. It puts more stress on the brain and leads to more sympathetic dominance (i.e., fight-flight-freeze-fawn response). When you're living in a perpetual fight-flight-freeze-fawn state due to emotional and physiological stressors, it is very hard to access your prefrontal cortex (the part of the brain responsible for

THE COPING MECHANISMS THAT KEPT YOU SAFE

impulse control and healthy decision-making) to make intentional changes. That's why you must address stress first by digging down to the root cause of the behavior. You must identify your need for comfort and figure out what core beliefs are tripping you up, leading you to seek out the instant gratification of a dopamine hit.

Making changes that stick requires executive function skills. Executive function skills include inhibitory control (the ability to think before you act), working memory (being able to focus on the task at hand while also thinking ahead to the next step), and cognitive flexibility (being able to switch from one task to another as plans change). Basically, executive function is how we manage procedures of day-to-day tasks while still rolling with the punches the day can bring. The more stressed and disconnected you are from the root cause of your issue, the harder it is to access executive function skills to make and sustain changes.

I had to draw on executive function recently when, during the peak heat of an East Texas summer, our air conditioning decided to give out. The same week, our garage door malfunctioned and needed repairs. The extra tasks of calling companies and scheduling services completely threw me off my schedule. I needed to adapt and be flexible, but the stress of scheduling repairs (and the exorbitant costs) brought out a desire for my old friend: Freeze Mode. I wanted to hide away and eat crunchy snack foods. To my overwhelmed brain, that seemed like the right choice.

However, because I've spent many years instilling habits that help my brain function more optimally in times of stress, I was able to pursue activities that helped me manage my stress in a more health-promoting way for long-term support. I loaded up on biblical truth during my morning reading time. I shared my disappointment with my husband instead of shutting him out. I made brain-boosting meals (and got creative to avoid overheating the house with the oven), and I stuck to my movement practice that helps move my body through stress. We even tried out some new restaurants using gift cards I (surprise!) found in my wallet.

Learning to change habits requires doing something difficult in the short-term that will benefit you in the long-term. However, until you have learned healthy emotional regulation, addressed your trauma and thought patterns, and begun to observe your behaviors (your old friends and any faulty core beliefs) with curiosity, it will be difficult to access your prefrontal cortex and executive function skills for impulse control.

As you process these patterns, you can start training your brain to change through the replacement method. That means that instead of completely quitting your habit, you replace it with something else you want. This way, you're slowly changing your habits in a way that doesn't disrupt your lifestyle and create more stress. This could look like

- reaching for your Bible instead of your phone first thing in the morning
- choosing dark chocolate and almonds instead of your nightly handful of candy or cookies
- opting for fruit-infused sparkling water or kombucha instead of your evening glass of wine
- having nutrient-dense snacks on hand instead of going through the drive-through for a 3:00 p.m. pick-me-up
- putting yourself to bed rather than watching another episode when you find yourself falling asleep on the couch
- meeting a friend at a nearby park for a walk-and-talk date rather than meeting for breakfast or lunch

THE COPING MECHANISMS THAT KEPT YOU SAFE

My client, Ben, who worried he was a food addict, found that he needed to replace his typical carb-heavy breakfast for one with more protein. He swapped his lunchtime soda for a seltzer. That led to sustained energy and reduced cravings the rest of the day. Are there any swaps you, like Ben, might make that would be more nourishing for you—mentally, physically, or spiritually? The replacement method allows you to create stress-supportive solutions that also support your health goals.

One of my favorite reminders of the power of replacement comes from the apostle Paul:

> Since, then, you have been raised with Christ, set your hearts on things above, where Christ is, seated at the right hand of God. Set your minds on things above, not on earthly things. For you died, and your life is now hidden with Christ in God.
> COLOSSIANS 3:1-3, NIV

When life is overwhelming and I'm struggling to send my old friends away, it helps me to remember that the battle I face isn't one I face alone. While my old friends try to convince me that the only comfort available to me is that of my own design, Scripture reminds me that I can set aside my faulty beliefs. I can walk in the freedom of my true identity because I am a wholly redeemed "new creation" (2 Corinthians 5:17).

I hope this truth brings comfort to you as well. Instead of putting on the old self and hanging out with your old friends, you can set your mind on the promise that you are being renewed in the image of your Creator every day. Even as you struggle with your daily habits.

Change and the Neurodivergent Brain

Neurodivergent is a nonmedical term describing the neurobiological differences in brains that receive and process information differently. It's often used to describe those who have been diagnosed with conditions such as autism, ADHD, and dyslexia, to name a few. The descriptor Highly Sensitive Person (HSP) is also believed to fit in this category. Some people consider bipolar disorder and other mental illnesses to exhibit neurodivergent brain patterns.

Whereas a *convergent* thinking pattern, common in those with neurotypical brain function, "brings together information that focuses on solving a problem, especially one that has a single, correct solution,"[2] a neurodivergent thinking pattern develops ideas in different directions, completely outside the box, or all at once. Because of this difference in thinking, those of us in the neurodivergent category can struggle even more with making habit changes. We may struggle with executive function and staying on task. Or we may become more easily overwhelmed by stress, which overloads our ability to problem solve.

If this is you, know that there is nothing wrong with you. Your brain simply works differently, so you may need a different approach to goal setting when it comes to changing bad habits. Start with one small habit change instead of addressing everything at once (I know that's not as exciting). Remind yourself that setbacks are part of life. Take extra care to support your nervous system and manage stress. It might take you a little bit longer than your neurotypical-brained friend to make changes, but you can make changes stick! For additional information and guidance, check out my friend Dr. Tamara Rosier's book *Your Brain's Not Broken*.

MAKING THE MIND-BODY CONNECTION

Here are two activities I use to help my clients deal with cravings and impulses when they hit:

THE COPING MECHANISMS THAT KEPT YOU SAFE

- **Perform a HEART check.** If you find yourself fighting the urge to engage in a habit you don't think is beneficial for you, pause what you're doing and take a deep breath. Check in with yourself to identify the emotion. Use the HEART acronym and ask yourself, *Am I: Hurting? Exhausted? Angry? Resentful? Tense?* Then ask, *Am I seeking comfort through this habit, or am I seeking stimulation from dopamine? Can I distinguish the difference?*

  We often seek comfort when we're experiencing one of the unpleasant emotions from the HEART check. Or we may be bored and in search of a quick dopamine boost for the brain. Even if you can't identify the emotion, that's okay. The goal of a HEART check is not necessarily to make sense of the why behind your behavior in the moment but to practice observing your response nonjudgmentally, which promotes self-compassion rather than self-criticism.

- **Practice havening.** This is a mind-body technique that uses sensory input (such as distraction, touch, and eye movements) to increase delta waves in the brain, which bring a state of calm. It has also been found to boost neurotransmitters such as serotonin and dopamine, which is often what we seek when we engage with our old coping mechanisms. There are three ways you can do this: rubbing your hands together, using your hands to rub your upper arms, or gently rubbing your face with your first three fingers, starting from center of nose and moving out to cheeks. For this exercise, we'll practice the first option.

  When the desire for your patterned behavior hits, take a deep breath in through your nose and exhale through your mouth. On the next inhale, rub your hands together and slowly exhale. Do this for a few rounds, then pause and check in with yourself. The goal of this activity is to create a sense of calm so you can evaluate the need for the behavior. It may decrease the desire, but if it doesn't, it still allows your body to respond from a state of peace instead of reacting from a state of stress. Do as many rounds as you'd like, or move to the other two movements, using your hands on your upper arms or touching your cheeks.

8

UNBLOCKING YOUR FEELINGS

Because of my label of bipolar disorder, I haven't always felt safe to feel my feelings. Throughout adolescence and early adulthood, my feelings weren't validated except as symptoms of my labels. According to experts, I was either depressed and experiencing symptoms of depression, or I was manic and experiencing symptoms of mania. When unpleasant feelings popped up, they were pathologized, medicated, and explained away with statements like, "It's just the chemicals in your brain needing support. When a diabetic's pancreas isn't producing enough insulin, they receive insulin. It's no different for mental illness."

The oversimplification invalidated very real feelings and pain, but I nodded my head, picked up the prescription, and shut the door on feeling anything. Even after experiencing a traumatic manic episode before my initial diagnosis of bipolar disorder, I was never given space to sort out what occurred. Despite being given a completely new identity, I had little support to process what it meant.

By suppressing my feelings as much as possible, I minimized the chance of experiencing negative symptoms that could be misconstrued as "mania" or "depression." Ignoring feelings kept me out of the doctor's office. If I powered through and stuck to my schedule of overactivity, I wouldn't have to deal with any unpleasant feelings that got in the way of the routine. Unless, of course, like a faulty pressure cooker, they exploded because of my repeated attempts to suppress them.

It wasn't until I sought out counseling in my forties that my trauma therapist Millie discovered I didn't even know how to name my feelings. This was a huge revelation because I was someone who felt everyone's feelings. I cared deeply—and too much—about everything. I had even been labeled "overly emotional" at one point. Yet, I couldn't put a name to my feelings. Apparently, *scattered* isn't a feeling. *Busy* isn't a feeling either. News to me!

Realizing I didn't trust my feelings or their expression helped me understand why I blocked them. I learned that I couldn't experience one feeling while I was simultaneously preoccupied with suppressing all the others. Which is why I had concluded that it was safer to suppress and stifle strong feelings—it was my attempt to avoid being labeled "mentally unstable." It was definitely not safe to feel my feelings.

I believe this dynamic of avoiding difficult feelings is all too common when we carry a label, regardless of what kind of label it is. The label creates a narrative (or confirms a faulty core belief) that our feelings are somehow dangerous, so we don't allow ourselves to process them. For those of us with labels, feelings are often not to be trusted. However, when we spend years in fear of our feelings and choose to block them, it creates problems that complicate our ability to heal.

The Problem with Blocking Feelings

Feelings are subjective pieces of information we receive subconsciously in response to the world around us. They're subjective because how we feel about something depends on our personal experiences, our past, and how our nervous system is responding to our current environment. It's important to distinguish between emotions and feelings. While they're often used interchangeably, they're actually different. "An *emotion* is a physiological experience (or state of awareness) that gives you information about the world," writes social science researcher Karla McLaren. "And a *feeling* is your conscious awareness of the emotion itself."[1] In other words, the emotion is automatic, and the feeling is the sensation that brings it to our attention.

Blocking feelings is a problem because it shuts out valuable information about our safety in the world, negatively impacts our physical health, and prevents us from having healthy relationships—with others, ourselves, and God.

Blocking feelings shuts down protective alerts. I recently asked my middle child, who is still in elementary school, why he thinks it's good to notice feelings. "Our feelings are there to protect us," he said. He's right! Ever had a "gut feeling" about something that turned out to be spot on? I know I have. Whether it's a subtle prickling on the back of my neck or an obvious sense of nervousness, this feeling has gotten me out of dangerous situations. On one occasion, I asked a store security guard to walk me to my car when I noticed a man was following me. It worked. As soon as the stranger saw me with the guard outside the store, he darted off.

Blocking feelings negatively impacts physical health. If we block feelings long enough, it creates stress. And because of our strong mind-body connection, that stress impacts our bodies. Prolonged stress can lead to increased production of stress hormones such as cortisol, which is needed to meet the demands of short-term stress but creates inflammation over the long-term. The stress of suppressing emotions can lead to increased blood sugar output, which is damaging to cellular function. There is a growing school of thought that fascia (the soft connective tissue that surrounds muscles, bones, and organs) is loaded with sensory receptors that respond to our emotional distress by storing that stress. A popular saying in massage therapy is, "The issues are in the tissues," which means that everything your brain refuses to process, your body chooses to store.

Blocking feelings makes it difficult to connect with others. Sooner or later, suppressed feelings will take a toll on a relationship. For example, if I feel disappointed because my husband didn't pick up an item from the grocery store on his way home from work, I may choose to squash that disappointment because I don't want to create an argument. But by stuffing the disappointment, I increase the likelihood that the next time I'm disappointed, I'll remember this grocery store disappointment and add a dose of resentment on top. Over time, accumulated disappointment and resentment can turn into bitterness. Then it's only a matter of time until a more explosive argument will occur. Simply sharing my disappointment as it arises prevents an escalation of other feelings and a bigger argument. And sharing my feelings, even when they're difficult, contributes to the health of our relationship by increasing vulnerability and intimacy.

Blocking feelings makes it difficult to connect with ourselves. When we block our feelings, we miss the signals our bodies are sending to ask for support. So many feelings start off as felt sensations of the body. Remember how I said the gut sends more signals to the brain than the brain does to the gut? Getting butterflies in your stomach before a social event is your body's way of letting you know you're anxious or excited. Perhaps you're in a hurry as

The Feeling Wheel

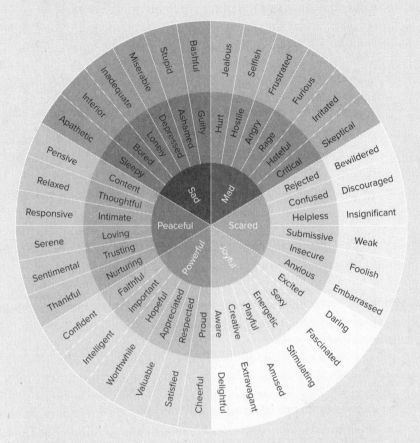

Have you heard of the feeling wheel? Originally developed by Dr. Gloria Willcox in 1982,[2] the feeling wheel has been variously adapted over the years, but most versions look something like a pie chart divided into three concentric circles, with each circle out from the middle subdivided into increasingly specific feelings.[3]

The inner circle lists six primary emotions: *joyful, powerful, peaceful, sad, mad,* and *scared*. In the second concentric circle, each of the six primary emotions are elaborated on with more specific feeling descriptors. For example, the primary emotion *sad* includes the feelings *guilty, ashamed, depressed, lonely, bored,* and *sleepy.* And it is the same for pleasant primary emotions such as *joyful*, which is broken down into feeling words such as *excited, sexy, energetic, playful, creative,* and *aware.* The third concentric circle then lists even more specific words for each word in the second circle. Being able to see such a wide range of feelings can be a helpful way to check in with yourself and identify what you're feeling, especially if you never felt safe expressing your feelings growing up, or if you experienced over-pathologizing of your feelings due to a mental health label.

you get ready for an event and so you're ignoring any feelings of anxiety—but your body alerts you through those belly flutters. If you ignore the sensations, they get stronger. For example, I feel buzzy and shaky before I speak at an event. If I don't pause and acknowledge my anxiety, that buzzy, shaky feeling will lead me to talk too fast and skip over important pieces of information at the beginning of my presentation—which happened recently when I forgot to introduce myself or say anything about who I am or what I do until about halfway through a presentation.

Blocking feelings makes it difficult to connect with our heavenly Father. When you are trying to connect with God through reading your Bible or prayer, blocking feelings is the equivalent of saying, "I'm fine." Just as that answer has become meaningless in day-to-day interactions and prevents deeper connections with others, it also prevents depth in your spiritual life and connection with God. Without access to your feelings, prayer and Bible reading will soon feel like you're just going through the motions, checking a box on your to-do list. Having access to your feelings is essential for growing in an intimate relationship with the one who created you and longs to have a real relationship with you.

Blocking feelings disrupts the human experience in virtually every area of life. Although choosing to suppress feelings and power through in survival mode may feel like safety in the short-term, it creates problems in the long-term that we'll have to overcome to heal. In order to flip the script and support the natural process, we must learn to normalize feelings instead.

Normalizing Feelings

To normalize feelings is simply to see them as, well, *normal*. By acknowledging and accepting them, we increase our awareness of how our brains and bodies are constantly sending us alerts. When we connect with our feelings instead of pushing them away, we are better able to regulate the ones that feel more intense than others. I once interviewed a therapist on my podcast who challenged me not to categorize feelings as bad or good. She pointed out that all feelings give us valid information, but the degree of comfort or discomfort the feelings give us depends on what kind of information the feelings are trying to convey.

Feelings of happiness and joy are much more comfortable to experience. Feelings of fear, anger, sadness, or disgust might cause more discomfort. Just as not all stress is bad, even the most unpleasant feelings aren't bad. But the degree to which we feel them strengthens their impact—positive or negative—on our well-being. Fear is a familiar feeling for the HPA axis (our internal alert system that tells our bodies to produce stress chemicals), and it is often there to tell us to change direction. Unfortunately, the felt sense of fear we experience might also be connected to past negative experiences or beliefs. So even if fear is trying to be protective, it can lead us away from legitimate and healthy opportunities for growth.

Checking in with an unpleasant emotion to determine its purpose can be a helpful way to normalize the resulting feeling. This starts with noticing the feeling and naming what the feeling is there for. For example, if you're fearful about an upcoming doctor's appointment, notice it. "I'm experiencing the feeling of fear right now. I'm fearful about my doctor's appointment." When I do this, I remind myself that it's okay to experience fear. Just giving myself that reminder is enough to normalize the feeling and accept it.

You can stop right there if you want, or you can take normalizing the feeling one step further by asking, "Is this feeling based on my current state or a past experience?" And the response might be, "I'm feeling fearful, because I had a rushed morning that didn't go as I planned, and I'm afraid of another unexpected outcome that will ruin my day." Or, "I'm feeling fearful because my friend went to a similar appointment and was diagnosed with cancer." Those are both valid fears! And they both have a purpose. In this case, the purpose of fear is driven by your HPA axis to get you to make a choice about how to deal with your fear: You can go to the doctor's appointment, or you can skip it. Your fear is based on your body's need to survive by avoiding potential threats. In either scenario, you have current and past experiences that suggest this appointment could be a threat, so your body alerts you with the sensation of fear to get you to escape the threat.

When we make it a habit to check in with our feelings and to become more familiar with them, we increase our mindfulness, which if you remember from chapter 3, increases self-compassion and partnership. It keeps us away from self-bullying and judgment. In my office, where I meet with clients, I have a printed copy of a feeling wheel and an emotion-sensation wheel. I use them when I sense that a client hasn't been allowed to feel feelings, has spent a lot of time in survival mode, or has been living in a pattern of chronic stress. Asking them to identify three specific feelings or sensations from the wheels enables them to share what they may not be allowing themselves to feel. When the unpleasant feelings want to take over and protect us too much (such as trying to get us to avoid the routine doctor's appointment), validating our feelings empowers us to choose our next step mindfully and intentionally rather than defaulting to fear or suppressing our feelings.

The more we normalize our feelings, the better we can care for our own needs. We can become more aware of what triggers us and why. And we can create the conditions in which it is safe for us to feel and learn to address unpleasant feelings before they build up.

Getting Acquainted with the God Who Feels

If normalizing feelings and understanding your wide array of feelings is scary for you, I understand. It has been extremely difficult for me to feel comfortable with feeling. But over the years, as I've dug deep into my own vortex of suppressed feelings, God has been so kind to show me evidence of his own feelings in Scripture, through stories of Jesus in the Gospels and through expressions of God's own emotions in passages from the Psalms, Isaiah, and Zephaniah. It gives me great comfort to know that I serve a God who also experiences a kaleidoscope of feelings. Here are some of my favorite reminders:

- *Anger.* Jesus expressed anger when he went to the Temple and saw merchants profiting from selling animals for sacrifice and exploiting the disadvantaged who could afford only pigeons. "Jesus entered the temple and drove out all who sold and bought in the temple, and he overturned the tables of the money-changers and the seats of those who sold pigeons. He said to them, 'It is written, "My house shall be called a house of prayer," but you make it a den of robbers'" (Matthew 21:12-13).

- *Grief.* Upon hearing the news of Lazarus's death, Jesus "was deeply moved in his spirit and greatly troubled" (John 11:33). Later, the text says, "Jesus wept" (John 11:35).

- *Dread and agony.* Just before his arrest and crucifixion, Jesus acknowledged his dread of what lay ahead when he prayed, "Father, if you are willing, remove this cup from me" (Luke 22:42). He was so overwhelmed by what he was about to endure that the stress manifested itself physically: "And being in agony he prayed more earnestly; and his sweat became like great drops of blood falling down to the ground" (Luke 22:44).

- *Compassion.* "For the LORD will vindicate his people and have compassion on his servants" (Psalm 135:14). The Lord feels compassion for his children when they're mistreated.

- *Empathy.* Jesus can feel our normal human feelings with us, because he's experienced them himself. "Surely he has borne our griefs and carried our sorrows" (Isaiah 53:4).

- *Joy.* Your Creator experiences joy over you. "He will rejoice over you with gladness; he will quiet you by his love; he will exult over you with loud singing" (Zephaniah 3:17).

God can handle your big feelings. He can handle your scattered brain. When your feelings seem bigger than the container you have to carry them in, he is standing by with a storage tank that never reaches capacity. He sees you, and he understands what you're going through. I love this promise from the psalmist, who says to God, "You've kept track of my every toss and turn through the sleepless nights, Each tear entered in your ledger, each ache written in your book" (Psalm 56:8, MSG). Your tears are precious to him, even when you feel ashamed that they're revealing your inner state, again.

Feelings are ever-changing, but God isn't. He is always true to his character, and he invites you to share all of yourself with him—even the feelings that you haven't figured out yet. Others may have shamed you for your feelings and tried to squelch them, or led you to believe you were "too much," but your heavenly Father doesn't view you that way. He is never too busy to listen to you, and he longs for you to bring your whole self to him—complicated feelings and all. Allow yourself to feel them. You and all your big feelings are safe with him.

MAKING THE MIND-BODY CONNECTION

The Examen or Daily Examen is a prayer of reflection developed by St. Ignatius in the sixteenth century to help us recognize God's presence in the events and experiences of an ordinary day. It's a way to check in with yourself at the end of a long day—to bring all your feelings to a God who "gets you," and to allow your feelings to draw you closer to him. When you become aware of your feelings, you can be more aware of how the Holy Spirit is moving in your life. The Examen typically involves five steps.

1. *Become aware of God's presence.* Review your day—morning, afternoon, and evening—in partnership with the Holy Spirit, who lives within you. Ask him to help you see each event and experience of your day through his eyes.

2. *Reflect with gratitude.* Recall any moments that made you smile and filled you with thankfulness. Consider the people you encountered and conversations you had, the beauty you noticed, the gifts of grace or comfort you received. In what ways was God present in each of those things? How did God move with you throughout your day?

3. *Notice feelings that popped up during your day.* Observing without judgment, identify the different feelings you experienced throughout the day. (If you struggle to name any emotions, consider using the feeling wheel, which you can find on page 119.) Did you feel frustration, sorrow, grief, joy, happiness, hope? What might God have been saying to you through these feelings? Ask God to speak into all the feelings you experience.

4. *Choose one part of your day to pray about.* Ask the Holy Spirit to point out one aspect of your day to focus on. Is there something you need to process further? Is there a feeling you're suppressing, a relationship or situation you're avoiding? Did you catch yourself checking out or trying not to feel at any point during the day? Ask God to help you remain present to your feelings even when you feel like shutting down or compartmentalizing them.

5. *Prepare for tomorrow.* Ask God to prepare your heart for what tomorrow holds. Take note of any feelings that arise when you consider what's ahead. Ask for boldness to enter a new day with a new set of feelings. Ask for peace and joy and gratitude to be an ever-present comfort and reminder that God is with you through the rise and fall of every feeling.

9

LOOKING FOR A MAGIC FIX

Imagine yourself in the following scenario. Over a period of three or four months, you begin to experience mysterious symptoms—a marked decrease in energy, intermittent insomnia, sudden cravings for sweets, and irritability. You feel like something isn't right, so you schedule an appointment with your practitioner to receive an evaluation and hopefully some answers. Your practitioner listens to your concerns, agrees that something might be off, and runs some routine lab work. When you return for your follow-up appointment, your practitioner sighs and says, "The good news is that all your blood levels are in the normal reference range. The bad news is you're just getting older. These things happen. Come back next year, and we'll run the labs again."

How would you feel? Probably invalidated and defeated, right?

Unfortunately, this is an all-too-common scenario experienced by my clients, and one I've experienced myself. When I was in college and struggling to find the right medication for my mental stability, I longed to be diagnosed with hypothyroidism. I wanted a medical explanation that would explain and justify my weight gain and fatigue. I wanted a pill to fix me. I wanted a concrete diagnosis based on labs, not a theoretical diagnosis based on symptoms. Unfortunately, my labs always came back "normal," even though I felt anything but normal. It wasn't until much later, when I understood the gut-brain connection, that I was able to make sense of why I'd struggled the way I had. Functional medicine—which focuses on finding interconnected patterns that create imbalances—helped me identify the root causes of my symptoms.

Now let's continue with our scenario. After hearing from your practitioner that you're fine (despite not feeling fine), you seek out support from an alternative practitioner you follow on social media who offers an exclusive program for those willing to pay for it. You spend a couple thousand dollars in lab work not covered by insurance, start taking fifteen different nutritional supplements, and begin a strict elimination diet that's free of gluten, dairy, corn, soy, sugar, alcohol—and all joy. You're determined to do everything you can to address your symptoms, but you begin to stress so much about doing the right things or missing a step that your symptoms get worse instead of improving.

Now what do you do?

Unfortunately, this, too, is a scenario often experienced by my clients. While I love helping others address root causes and find assistance from targeted supplementation and dietary changes, the alternative method can sometimes send people on an endless quest to find *the* root cause of their issues, as if uncovering one missing puzzle piece will solve all their problems. Sometimes this approach helps, but other times a very rigid, rule-based journey to health ends up creating nothing but more chronic stress.

I call this the never-ending journey to find a magic fix. It's a pursuit that typically begins with curiosity and self-advocacy but can sometimes escalate into a fixation for some of us. We become preoccupied with our health journeys to the point that we're obsessed with finding answers, and that obsession becomes a stressor—especially when the answers elude us. And when that stress is ongoing and chronic, it can lead to inflammation and negative health outcomes, both emotionally and physiologically. Which means our pursuit of the magic fix only adds to our stress.

When Looking for Solutions Adds to Your Stress

This stressful pursuit of a magic fix isn't new. Diet culture has been loud and in our faces since early in the twentieth century through magazines, then radio and television ads. Growing up, I tried all the diets in hopes of fixing not just my body's appearance but my satisfaction with my body's appearance. It didn't take very many crash diets for me to realize that adhering to a strict diet was relatively easy, but learning to accept the shape of my body at any weight or size wasn't. I never found the magic size or number on the scale. I only grew unhappier and more stressed out about my body.

Fast-forward to today and social media has only amplified diet culture and body dissatisfaction. We now have 24-7 access to news cycles and influencer posts driven by an algorithm catered to our interests. So if searching for health solutions is important to you, you'll likely find every available magical fix showing up in your feed through sponsored ads and influencers who claim to have been where you are. I'm not one to blame everything on social media, but I do think the age of information overload compounds the phenomenon of health obsession. Maybe it's just the algorithm feeding my health coaching interests, but these days I see less interest in dieting for body modification and more interest in biohacking—optimizing human health, performance, and longevity through the latest research and tools. There's always a new study, device, or technique promising to change the expression of our genes, increase our longevity, and decrease our health symptoms. But chasing every new thing can be both pricey and stressful. At worst, it can take us completely off course, leaving us feeling worse than before. Just ask my client Robin.

Robin reached out to me for genetic testing because she was concerned she had a genetic SNP (single nucleotide polymorphism) called MTHFR.[1] After reading about it on a social media post and identifying with some of the associated symptoms, she immediately started down the rabbit hole of blogs, research articles, and Facebook groups. She learned that folic acid is toxic to those who have this genetic SNP because they can't convert folic acid to folate, its most bioavailable form. She eventually became so paranoid about this genetic "mutation" that she stayed up late most nights researching, which caused her to miss out on supportive rest. In addition to worsening her physical symptoms, her fatigue and preoccupation left her feeling irritable and eventually created tension between her and her husband.

When I met with Robin, I had to gently explain that while there is a genetic SNP called MTHFR that makes it difficult for the body to function optimally, there are millions of other SNPs we don't know as much about. Learning about one SNP might be helpful for understanding presenting symptoms and struggles, but there is still a lot we don't understand about how environmental factors influence our gene expression. I needed her to see how getting wrapped up in chasing one magic solution might be causing her more stress and unanswered questions.

Focusing too much on one thing as *the* answer to all our problems can also cause us to lose focus on the basics, such as getting good rest, eating nutritious food, moving our bodies, and practicing mindfulness. And the most important basic that is commonly overlooked when pursuing the magic fix is this: learning to listen to our own unique bodies.

The Wisdom of Listening to Your Body

Allow me to remind you of something that may seem obvious but is often overlooked: *You are the only person in your body.* You are the only person *with* your body. Nobody else has the exact same body as you—not even if you're an identical twin. God has designed your body to speak to you via symptoms, and there is wisdom in listening to the signals it sends you. When you learn to listen to your body and appreciate its design, even the search for a new and shiny magic fix may grow less appealing.

Tuning in to the needs of your body requires at least two things: You must create safety for your nervous system, and you must partner with your body.

Create Safety for Your Nervous System

As you may recall from chapter 4, God created your body as a protective agent to alert you to danger. If your body is constantly receiving signals of incoming threats, whether real or perceived, it will prioritize survival over long-term healing. That can create unsafety in the nervous system. The body won't heal in a chronic state of sympathetic (fight-flight-freeze-fawn) activation. That's how a chronic pursuit of wellness via a magic fix can come at the expense of finding a parasympathetic (rest-and-digest) state. For those of us who have struggled with our health for a long time, learning how to activate a parasympathetic state may feel like learning a second language. It's unfamiliar when you've been living off stress chemicals. Even though these alert signals in your body want to keep your Worst-Case Scenario Brain ready for action, it is possible to create safety.

Creating safety with your nervous system takes time and intention—and it requires nourishment. I often challenge my clients to ask themselves in the morning, "What does my body need for nourishment today?" Remember, nourishment includes *anything* needed for health, not just food. So for some people, getting the nourishment they need may mean skipping the early morning workout and choosing a slow wake-up instead. For others, it might mean taking a morning prayer walk—rather than sitting still in prayer—to release excess stress. Maybe it's changing lunch or dinner plans so you can save energy for a demanding task. Perhaps instead of hurriedly drinking a smoothie in the car on the way to work, you get up a little earlier so you can sit down for a warming breakfast. Or maybe you unfollow some social media accounts that make you feel like you should be doing more.

Here's another question I encourage my clients to ask: "Does my current pace of life contribute to a felt sense of safety or a felt sense of stress in my nervous system?" For example, does your body feel safe to heal? Do you make time for purposeful relaxation activities, or do you push yourself until you crash? One way to check into this is by reviewing your daily activities. What part of your day is dedicated to slowing down and getting still (without doomscrolling on your phone)? Is your schedule so crammed that you never have time to just sit and breathe? These are all indicators that your body may not feel safe to heal.

I don't ask about your schedule to shame you about your pace of life. I, too, am a chronic over-scheduler, and I like staying busy. But when I finally dug down deep and got curious about my patterns, I found that at the root of my need for busyness was fear. I feared that if I slowed down too much, I would crash—that my former depression would rear its nasty head. My busyness kept me going at a pace that blunted all emotions as well as all warning signals to slow down.

Your body needs to feel safe to slow down and heal. A good way to do that is to take small segments of time during the day, and longer chunks on the weekend, to support your nervous system through something that is calming for you.

Partner with Your Body

Here's another thing that may seem obvious but is often overlooked: *Your body is a temple, not a remodeling project.* Your body is a masterpiece of God's human architecture, not a storage unit for your self-improvement plans. Maybe that comes off a little cheesy to you, but it's true. When you choose to partner with your body instead of focusing on incessant remodeling projects for it, you are more aware of its innate purpose and design.

Too often on our health journeys, we do what we think we need instead of asking our bodies what they actually need. To complicate matters, we let other people tell us what's best for our bodies—especially when they promise a quick fix—without ever once consulting with our bodies' Master Architect about what our bodies need to feel good. We tend to allow other humans into the remodeling process before we invite our Creator (the one who designed us) into it. However, when we partner with our bodies, we choose to be present *in them* instead of trying to fix them with the next new thing.

To be present in your body is to experience embodiment. Embodiment enables you to feel connected to your body and the sensations it gives you. It is a way to partner with your body and listen to it, even when you'd prefer to keep blazing forward with your hands over your ears. When you practice embodiment, you choose mindfulness, curiosity, and self-compassion about the symptoms your body is sending to you.

The idea of embodiment and partnering with the body was a new idea for my client Courtney, who had tried many magic fixes to beat her autoimmunity into submission. She'd been to many practitioners before me, and they always told her that, due to the nature of her various autoimmune diseases, her body "was attacking itself."[2] I urged her to flip the script and change the question from "Why is my body attacking me?" to "Why is my body working so hard to protect me, and how can I help it to feel safe?" That reframing transformed everything she did going forward. She adopted an approach of partnership over punishment and bullying, and she experienced many positive health outcomes as a result.

Searching endlessly for a magic fix may feel like you're addressing the root cause, but when it takes you away from listening to

Indicators That You're Choosing Partnership over Punishment

Listed below are several examples of ways to check in and partner with your body. Place a check mark next to any that are true for you. And give yourself grace if you aren't able to check any. Simply consider what might be preventing you from choosing to partner with, rather than punish, your body.

- ☐ You allow yourself to feel and name your feelings without judgment.
- ☐ You ask your body what it needs for support.
- ☐ You rest when you need to rest.
- ☐ You accept that things don't always go as planned, and that's okay.
- ☐ You give yourself grace when your own expectations aren't met.
- ☐ You connect with your body regularly by checking in on it through breathing breaks.
- ☐ You've learned ways to quiet your inner critic.
- ☐ You make time in your schedule for rest and relaxation.

the needs of your body and partnering with it for safety, it only creates more added stress.

Your Body Is Not Your Enemy

Your body is an ally to partner with, not an enemy to battle. I understand that idea may be hard to accept, especially if you grew up receiving only negative messages about your body. When I work with female clients or speak to women's groups, I often ask them, "Growing up, did you ever hear positive messages about the human body from adults in your life?" Most women have to search really hard to find a memory of a positive message. What they heard instead were the negative things that needed to be fixed—and not just about body image and body modification, but about issues such as menstrual cramps, menstrual migraines, "the period flu," and all the aspects of womanhood. The complexity of the female body is almost always described as a burden, not a benefit. However, such body-talk flies in the face of what Scripture tells us about the inherent goodness of being created by God.

> "O Lord, what a variety of things you have made! In wisdom you have made them all."
> PSALM 104:24, NLT

> The Lord takes pleasure in all he has made!
> PSALM 104:31, NLT

> For we are his workmanship, created in Christ Jesus for good works, which God prepared beforehand, that we should walk in them.
> EPHESIANS 2:10

Your body is every bit as much a part of God's miraculous creation as the beautiful sunset you capture and post to your Instagram story or the expanse of the ocean that fills you with wonder. It's not selfish to be grateful for how you've been designed. It's not prideful to marvel in awe at all the things your body does to keep you alive every day. God's masterful design is on purpose just as you are here on purpose, for a purpose.

Reminder: *Your body is a temple, not a remodeling project.*

When you war against yourself in any capacity, you become your own enemy. You become your own stressor—emotionally and physiologically. But consider what Jesus says about your enemies: "Love your enemies and pray for those who persecute you" (Matthew 5:44).

I don't have any true enemies I can think of. I don't face persecution (keyboard warriors don't count). But if my greatest enemy is myself, and the person persecuting me is myself, I am called to respond in love. I am called to pray for my enemy, even when the enemy is me.

King David once prayed, "Though an army encamp against me, my heart shall not fear; though war arise against me, yet I will be confident" (Psalm 27:3). You may feel that you are your own enemy army, warring against yourself, and you have been for your entire life. But there is freedom. There is protection. There is safety. The bully within may be spewing lies and hatred, telling you that you aren't enough and that you can do more, but God is your shield and your refuge. He is the One True Thing you can trust, and his words about you are true. You bear the image of your Creator, and you have value just as you are, no matter what you're trying to fix.

You don't have to force yourself to believe in your inherent worth and value if you don't feel ready, but perhaps you can allow yourself to be present in the body you have. If you find the idea of loving your body difficult, you can start by appreciating its function and design. You can listen to the signals it sends you and commit to partnering with it going forward.

Your body is not your enemy. Your body is the vessel you've been given to live out your purpose. Step away from the quest for the magic fix and instead focus on listening to the needs of your body. You only have one.

MAKING THE MIND-BODY CONNECTION

The following activities are designed to help you learn to partner with your body and bring safety to it through intentional activation of the parasympathetic (rest-and-digest) state.

- **Legs up the wall meditation.** This is my favorite activity to do to restore safety to my body at the end of a long day, but it can be helpful anytime you need a minute to get back into your body. Try it at different times during the day throughout the week to see what works best for you, like after a workout, when you get home from work, or before bed.

    First, find a wall and sit down on the floor beside it. Gently swing or walk your legs up against the wall while simultaneously lowering your upper body to the floor, back lying securely on the ground. You can lie on a mat or blanket if that feels more supportive. Adjust your hips and backside so they are as close to the wall as is comfortable for you. Your legs can be straight against the wall or slightly bent if that's more comfortable. Rest your arms out to the sides, palms facing up or down. You can rest one hand on your belly and one on your chest for a more grounding experience.

    Practice breathing deeply into your belly, inhaling to fill your diaphragm with air and exhaling to let it all out. Another option is to do this while listening to your favorite worship song, one that fills you with gratitude and praise. Stay here for three to five minutes, or longer if you have time. The goal is to slow down and reconnect with your body and your Creator, practicing a parasympathetic state.

- **Gratitude and embodiment meditation.** This activity helps you to pay attention to the sensations your body gives you and to practice embodiment through gratitude for those body parts. You can practice this in any position you like, whether with legs up the wall, lying flat, or seated.

    As you take deep breaths in and out, do a body scan (such as the Head, Stomach, Chest, and Back exercise on page 21). As you breathe into various parts of your body, thank God for how your body has served you and protected you over time, even those parts you struggle with. For example, "Thank you, God, for my belly. I struggle to partner with my belly because of the discomfort it causes me, but I know your design is miraculous and some of my symptoms may be here to protect me in ways I don't yet understand. Please help me to tune in to and listen to my body's needs." I find it particularly grounding to think about my feet, and so I pray, "Thank you, God, for the support my feet provide me. Thank you for the miles they've walked me through and the miles they will carry me in the months and years ahead. Thank you for using my feet to take me out of harmful situations and onto paths that bring peace. Keep me grounded and rooted in your truth above all else."

PART 3

LEARN to address stress

IDENTIFY the root issues

ADD **VARIETY** TO YOUR DIET

EXERCISE your body and brain

I struggled with a chronic illness for over two decades before I learned the role that diet and nutrition play in my health—specifically, my brain health. When I speak to groups about fundamental nutrition concepts and the impact on the brain, the follow-up questions and messages I receive later tell me I'm not the only one who didn't know about the food-mood connection. What you eat creates building blocks for the trillions of cells in your body. But if you're like most people, you've never really paid attention unless you're on a diet to lose weight.

In part 3, we'll dig into your diet, but probably not in the way you might expect. I want to talk about *how* you eat, *why* you eat, and *what* you eat—and how that variety plays a role in creating safety for your nervous system. Adding variety to your diet through your mindset about food, the food itself, and your body image creates a foundation of health that every cell of your body picks up on. If you've ever felt intimidated and overwhelmed by all the nutrition advice out there, that's okay! We'll slowly and gently walk through the process of evaluating the role food plays in your life. Together, we'll untangle a lot, including things I wish someone had told me decades ago. I can't wait!

10

A BODY IN STRESS WON'T DIGEST

I can't attend a potluck without thinking about the time I overdosed on cherry pie.

I was seven, and apparently old enough to have free rein over what I ate. We were at a park in Tracy, California, where my dad was the pastor of the church hosting a picnic. As a rule-following preacher's daughter and firstborn, I typically did what was expected of me to keep up appearances. So I felt capable of assessing the food situation and serving myself. No problem there.

But I couldn't have anticipated the way the cherry pie would hit me. The doughy, glutenous crust combined with the sweet and tangy cherry pie filling was like a flavor burst for my taste buds and a light bulb for my brain. I remember so clearly that instant demand for more. Nobody was watching, so I took another piece. And another. And another. I joyfully rode the cherry pie high until later that night when I woke up with the worst stomachache. I spent a good bit of the night hugging the toilet and vowing to never eat cherry pie again. (Spoiler alert: I did.)

That didn't stop me from overdosing on fudge-dipped ice cream bars from a shop in the mall in fifth grade. Or from eating eight (*eight!*) Boston cream pie doughnuts one Sunday morning before the youth service started when I was fifteen. And it didn't keep me from blowing through an entire bag of Nacho Cheese Doritos on a fall hayride. Years later, as a teacher struggling to stay awake during the teacher in-service meetings we had right before school officially started, I couldn't keep my hands out of the candy basket filled with fun-size candy bars they laid at the center of every table. And I needed one Diet Coke or Dr Pepper every day of my adolescent and adult life until I was thirty-three.

I've always loved food, especially in sugar form—and the more, the better. Despite living with the luxury of having enough of it to keep me hooked, it never seemed to be enough. I always needed more.

As a result, from an early age I felt guilty for my indulgence. I tried cutting back. I went on all the crash diets of the 1990s, demonizing food groups and restricting intake to control my overconsumption urges. It never worked, so my inner drill sergeant yelled at me to make changes, and the cycle of indulge-diet-indulge continued.

It took a long time for me to restore a healthy relationship with food, beyond using it for momentary pleasure or restrictive dieting and counting calories. I knew food impacted how I felt emotionally, but I didn't realize how much my attitude toward food negatively impacted my mental health and relationship with my body. Peeling back the layers of that onion took a lot of time. As I progressed in my healing journey, this restored relationship with food played a transformational role in why I pursued training in integrative nutrition to help others with similar patterns.

When I first started my holistic health coaching business, I came up with the motto, "A body in stress won't digest." Even today, I repeat this at least once a session with my clients. This phrase informs everything I do, and I can't wait to share with you one of my greatest aha moments about nutrition: *How* and *why* you eat may matter more than *what* you eat.

How You Eat Impacts Your Digestion

Diet and fitness enthusiasts want you to believe that you are what you eat. And sure, I can partially get on board with that. On a cellular level, every nutrient consumed acts as food for the cell membrane and assists in either taking out the cellular trash or creating more of it. But in my research and my work with clients, I like to go one step further. *You are what you* think *about what you eat.* And beyond that, you are what your body can digest, utilize, and get past the cell membrane to create energy for the body. Even more importantly, the way your body digests food depends a great deal on what kind of stress you're currently facing.

We've already explored how our thoughts impact our health, so you've probably figured out that thoughts play a powerful role in digestion too. And they do. In fact, before digestion occurs in the gut, you experience the *cephalic phase of digestion*. The cephalic phase of digestion happens in your mind. When you smell a pleasing aroma, when you hear the oven timer ding, when you see the server approach your table with steaming plates, your body takes note. As you receive sensory input from your food, your body responds physically by preparing for digestion. There's even a cephalic phase insulin response, which occurs when your body prepares to secrete insulin in response to the thought of something sweet. The cephalic phase insulin response is believed to be important for regulating blood sugar after a meal.[1] How crazy is that?

Digestion is then optimized as you take your time to chew, breathe between bites (because you need oxygen to digest food), and savor the complex flavors hitting your tongue. The more complex the flavors, the more signals of satiety your body receives.

The digestive process is one of my favorite topics to cover with clients. Sorry not sorry—I get excited to talk about digestion! Here's why. Optimal digestion occurs when we give our bodies an optimal environment in which to digest. Eating in a state of stress is not an optimal environment. When the gut receives signals from the brain that we're in a state of fight-flight-freeze-fawn, it prioritizes survival over digestion. If survival is prioritized, then gastric emptying can be delayed, increasing stomachaches, indigestion, and gastrointestinal distress. In some cases, prioritizing survival means speeding things up, leading to quick emptying, such as diarrhea (so inconvenient, especially if you're stressed before something important, such as a presentation or job interview). This is why when I'm speaking at an event where a meal is provided to all attendees, I politely take a few bites or choose not to eat. I don't want to confuse my digestive response.

Knowing how stress impacts digestion, imagine what happens when you quickly consume fast food in your car. While I doubt anyone hates the enticing aroma of hot french fries in their passenger seat, not taking the time to savor and chew does the body a disservice. Even the concept of fast food can be a disservice. When you constantly eat whatever is convenient, on the go, in a hurry, in your car, you send a message to your body that due to an impending threat, there isn't time for proper nourishment.

When you're running late and frustrated with your kids about what they are eating (or not eating), you send that chemical stress message to every cell of your body. Your body responds out of protection by cuing the shutdown of digestion, because ancestrally speaking, there's no time to stop for a snack if you're being chased

A BODY IN STRESS WON'T DIGEST

by a saber-toothed tiger. Remember, your body responds to a real threat and a perceived threat the same way. To keep you safe, it activates protective mechanisms, such as increasing the stress hormone cortisol, spiking blood sugar, and decreasing digestive juices for the breakdown and absorption of nutrients.

One of my favorite ways to illustrate how the brain and body respond to food simultaneously is the milkshake study. In this study, participants were given a milkshake that contained 300 calories. However, one group was told that it was called "Sensishake," and it was only 140 calories, with zero fat and zero sugar. The other half of the group was told it was called "Indulgence," and that it was 620 calories and filled with all sorts of rich ingredients.

Before and after consuming the shakes, participants had their levels of ghrelin tested. Ghrelin is a hunger hormone that goes up when we're hungry and drops when we're full. It's the hormone that tells us it's time to eat. If you have a big meal, your ghrelin levels will drop because you are satiated. If you have a small meal or a snack, you will still be hungry, so you will still have higher levels of ghrelin.

Since both groups were given the exact same shake with the exact same ingredients and caloric value, it would stand to reason that it would be digested the exact same way. But what happened was pretty shocking for researchers. The group that drank the Indulgence shake had levels of ghrelin three times lower than the group that drank the Sensishake shake. The Indulgence group was overly stuffed, and the Sensishake group had a "flat" ghrelin response.[2]

Remember how I said you aren't *what* you eat, but you are what you *think* about what you eat? More research needs to be done beyond this one study, but isn't it fascinating to see just one of the ways mindset influences digestion?

Your relationship with food matters because what you think about food impacts how you digest your food. Chronic or acute stress before or during a meal disrupts digestion. But there's another piece to puzzling through a healthy food relationship. That piece is *why* you eat. Your beliefs about food and its purpose play a big role in your stress response.

Why You Eat Impacts Your Nervous System

Whether you realize it or not, your relationship with food and the way you view it provide important information for the autonomic nervous system through your felt sense of safety in the world.

It's not uncommon for me to encounter two types of clients in my coaching practice. Client A likes food rules and rigid guidelines. This type of client wants to know exactly what to eat to be healthy, and they don't worry about whether they enjoy it. They desire to see food as fuel alone and frown on phrases such as "emotional eating." Client B, on the other hand, has strong emotional ties to certain foods and eating habits. Food brings comfort and pleasure. This type of client wants to know what's best to eat, but they worry it won't really matter because their appetite is ruled by what they feel like eating in the moment.

How about you? Do you relate more to client A or client B?

This might surprise you, but these client types are strikingly similar. People who exhibit characteristics of client A want to do the right thing, but they aren't completely sure they can trust their bodies to naturally lead them toward healthy habits. And people who share characteristics of client B also want to do the right thing, but they aren't completely sure they can trust their bodies to lead them away from their emotional ties. They want the same thing. They want to be able to eat food that makes them feel satisfied and, ultimately, makes their bodies feel safe to function optimally.

So is it possible for food to be used as fuel, but also for comfort, pleasure, and celebration? My short answer: *Yes*. But I want to break this down a little more because this is where we often get tripped up on our health journeys, especially when we start having conversations about eating habits.

Any nutrition expert who tries to convince you that food is only for fuel is missing the bigger picture. We all know deep down that food is much more than fuel. If you've ever been on the receiving end of meals given after the loss of a loved one or birth of a child, you know this to be true. In this case, food is a form of love and care. Someone puts their energy into providing something you have no time or energy to provide yourself. It's not just fuel; it's a hug in a casserole dish.

Likewise, any nutrition expert who chastises those who eat for comfort or enjoyment is missing out as well. I can't imagine a world without celebratory meals. Holidays, birthdays, an evening with good friends—such rituals are essential to humanity. Even in the Old Testament, God ordained multiple feasts for the Jewish people to celebrate as a way to remember what he had done in their lives.

Your ancestors likely celebrated with feasts because a bountiful harvest was something to celebrate in the days when there were no grocery stores, much less grocery delivery. Even today, food tells your body that it doesn't need to worry because there is enough—enough nutrients to provide cellular energy; enough flavors and textures to provide satisfaction for a few hours; and enough nourishment to enter rest-and-digest mode, activating the parasympathetic state to bring resilience and relief to your nervous system.

For many, the way they view their plate reflects how they view the world and their safety in it. I routinely see clients with a disordered relationship to food as well as clients labeled with an eating disorder. For one of my clients with bulimia, food posed a potential danger or threat. Due to a past medical injury, she feared health interventions. Food was just one more thing needed for health that she wasn't sure she could trust. She became frightened of certain ingredients, and her body began to wither away.

For my client who experienced childhood sexual abuse, food offered protection. She told herself at a young age that if she ate enough to gain weight, her predators would no longer find her as appealing. When she revealed that to me, I couldn't stop the tears for the little girl who didn't feel safe in her body, so she created safety with food.

For my clients with mental illness or autoimmune diseases, there can be confusion about what foods will trigger their issues, or what foods are damaging to their gut. Food becomes a means to control their bodies, despite their deep fear that their bodies are falling apart on them.

When knowing what to eat or not eat becomes an emotional stressor on the body, the nervous system takes note. When food rules become a way to control life's chaos, the nervous system may see the act of eating as a threat instead of an activity to enter a rest-and-digest state.

Food is more than just fuel, and there are many reasons to eat beyond basic nutritional needs. When you understand those things, you can start to shift into a healthier relationship with food, built on a partnership with your body.

Restore Your Relationship with Food

There's one more piece to the food relationship puzzle we haven't addressed yet, and it might stir up stronger feelings. Here it is: To restore our relationship with food, we need to stop equating healthy eating habits with morality.

You're not a bad person if you eat a Snickers when you're sad.

You're not a bad person if you daydream about what you're going to eat at the restaurant tonight.

You're not a bad person if you prefer dark chocolate over asparagus (hi, I'm that person).

Just as there are different reasons for eating, different types of food serve different purposes. You have freedom to eat what's best for you. You don't have to berate yourself if you feel like you overindulged one night. Your body typically lets you know.

Your body will let you know if something is working for you or not. That's part of your design. When you intentionally tune in to your body's needs, listening to its symptoms and viewing nutrition as another way to gently partner with it, it's possible that you'll make different choices.

Shaming your body into change never gets you anywhere. But do you know what does set you on the right path? Consulting your body's architect. In fact, may I remind you of something really important that often gets missed?

God cares about your body.

You may think he doesn't care about a detail such as food, but he cares about how you receive sustenance and healing. He cares about how your nutrition supports your neurotransmitters because he designed the entire complex system to work that way. He knows when you're undereating and depriving yourself. God knows when you're overeating and not being mindful. He even knows how your stressed brain will prevent your body from digesting. "Better a small serving of vegetables with love than a fattened calf with hatred" wrote wise King Solomon (Proverbs 15:17, NIV). Even he knew that a body in stress won't digest.

God cares about your relationship with food, and even how your physical needs for sustenance are provided for. Perhaps you remember these words spoken by Jesus:

> Therefore I tell you, do not be anxious about your life, what you will eat or what you will drink, nor about your body, what you will put on. Is not life more than food, and the body more than clothing? Look at the birds of

the air: they neither sow nor reap nor gather into barns, and yet your heavenly Father feeds them. Are you not of more value than they?
MATTHEW 6:25-26

If God cares about how birds get fed, surely he cares about how you are fed, strict food guidelines or not.

Inviting your body's designer into the conversation can also be a way to increase compassion for yourself. You're not in this struggle alone. Restoring a healthy view of food in our current cultural climate is hard. For some, it's straight up anxiety inducing, and it can lead to food obsession and lack of trust in the needs of our own bodies. But as we established early on, food isn't our primary nourishment. Our primary nourishment—our relationships with God, others, and ourselves—sets the stage for how we receive our secondary nourishment.

When we eat in a relaxing environment and in a state of gratitude, we digest better. Even praying before a meal can support the rest-and-digest response of the nervous system and help us eat more slowly, giving our gut-brain connection time to communicate.

The nutrients in food matter a great deal to your overall health, but before you make any changes in your diet, I encourage you to take one small step first. Rethink *how* you eat before you consider *what* you eat. The way you eat provides your body with crucial information about your state of stress, because after all, a body in stress simply won't digest.

MAKING THE MIND-BODY CONNECTION

I encourage my clients to practice eating hygiene, which is just another way to describe mindful eating. The following practice is designed to

A BODY IN STRESS WON'T DIGEST

help you engage with all your senses while eating so you don't dissociate or get distracted during a meal, which hinders digestion.

- **Choose a meal you know will be the least stressful.** Allow at least twenty minutes for this meal. If you're a parent to young children, you may need to arrange for a babysitter and take yourself on a lunch date or do this during naptime. If your kids are school-aged, practice this during a lunch when they're at school. While we all love our kids, family mealtimes can be demanding and not the best time to use this practice.

- **Pause, breathe, and express gratitude.** Seat yourself comfortably for your meal. Before diving in, take a few deep breaths, maybe some rounds of 4-7-8 breathing (page 77). Say a prayer of gratitude for your meal and ask God to prepare your body for digestion. Look at your food and appreciate the aroma and appearance of it before you take your first bite.

- **Chew and notice.** As you begin eating, chew each bite at least twenty times. Notice the taste, texture, and smell of the food. How does it sound while you chew? Between bites, continue to take deep breaths to allow oxygen to help your body break down your food. If you need to drink, allow yourself no more than four ounces of water and sip slowly. Too much water during a meal interferes with digestion. Continue chewing and noticing the sensory input for a full twenty minutes.

- **Reflect.** How did this practice of mindful eating impact your feeling of fullness? Your satisfaction level? Commit to trying this practice during more meals throughout your week, as your schedule allows.

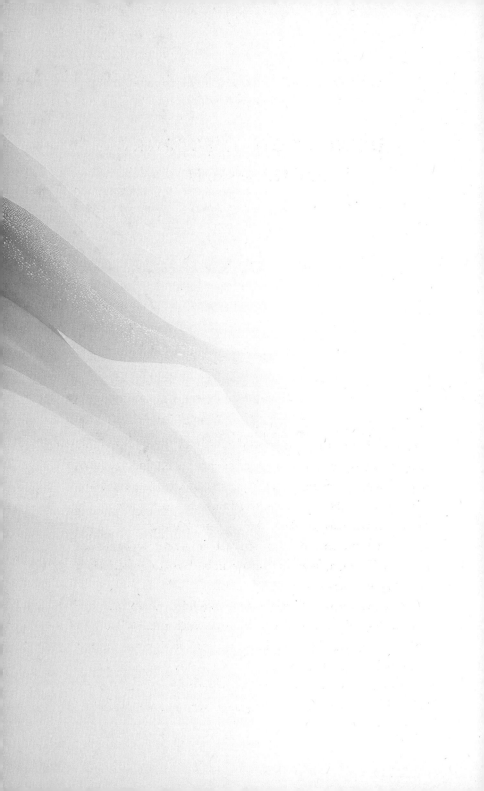

11

USING FOOD TO SUPPORT YOUR MOOD

"I'm really just here for a meal plan," Katie said. "I don't have time to figure this out myself, and I don't know which Instagram nutrition influencer is telling the truth. Just tell me what to eat and how to make it." As she sat in my office, arms crossed, it was clear my new client was exasperated by the concept of nutrition.

I smiled and nodded. "You're right, there are so many opinions out there. Trying to figure out what your body needs to feel its best can be pretty overwhelming."

"Exactly," she said, throwing her hands up in agreement. "I've done it all—paleo, keto, Whole30, vegan. Everything is fine for a little while, I guess. The only thing I haven't done is carnivore, and I just can't with all that meat!"

"How do you know when food is making you feel good?" I asked. "How do you know when you're getting everything you need?"

She frowned. "I don't know. When I just do a plan, I like it, and I definitely feel good. But then when I'm stressed or hungry or in a hurry, I go back to my Chick-fil-A and Cheez-Its. It takes so much effort to think about being healthy. I know I probably need more vegetables and less sugar, but it's hard to be consistent!"

Conversations like this one are on frequent replay in my office. Most of my clients want to eat better because they know they'll feel better. But the *how* of it all is overwhelming. It's hard to train your brain to try a new thing, especially if that new thing doesn't provide the instant reward (and MSG[1]) that a fried chicken sandwich does.

Perhaps you've noticed how the topic of nutrition tends to bring about a religious fervor that makes people zealots. Some vegans parade their cause like martyrs, while some carnivores post their muscles and fatty meat with the pride of Roman gladiators. All the experts believe their way of eating is the best, which leaves everyone else floundering in the deep end of a pool filled with good intentions and eventually giving up. As my clients often complain, it's so hard to know how to eat and be consistent! Especially when nutrition science always seems to be changing. We've gone from the experts saying, "Eat margarine because butter is bad for your heart," to the latest research indicating that margarine increases inflammation[2] and the *Journal of the American College of Cardiology* saying they "found no beneficial effects of reducing SFA intake [or saturated fat intake] on cardiovascular disease."[3]

To complicate matters more, while many of my clients are familiar with dieting for body modification purposes, addressing nutrition for whole body health is a foreign concept—until they find themselves diagnosed with a chronic condition and their doctor tells them to change their diet. Though the exact diet they should follow isn't always specified. And for those diagnosed with a mental health condition, nutrition is rarely discussed in the psychiatrist's office. After all, most are told their condition is due to a chemical imbalance. What does food have to do with that?

Actually, it has everything to do with it.

Allow me to introduce you to an entirely different way of looking at food. Food *is* mood, and I can't wait to explain why. When you begin to make the food-mood connection, it can be one of the most useful tools in your health journey.

Making the Food-Mood Connection

On the ever-growing list of "Things I Wish I Had Known When I Was First Diagnosed with Depression," the way food impacts mental well-being is close to the top. What we eat plays a significant role in how we feel. Neurotransmitters such as serotonin (known as the "happy" chemical messenger) and dopamine (the chemical messenger that supports motivation) are produced by nutrients in food. Even acetylcholine (the neurotransmitter that regulates vagus nerve function for your nervous system) is made from nutrients. As psychiatrist and nutrition expert Dr. Georgia Ede writes, "If you are short on certain nutrients, your neurons will not be able to manufacture all the neurotransmitters your brain needs to function properly."[4]

How and why you eat are crucial for developing a healthy relationship with food, but what you eat still matters for your body and brain. While it can be complicated to figure out what food is right for you, I believe there are three specific ways that food affects mood—through your gut microbiome, your blood sugar, and your nutrients. When you understand these three areas, you can learn how to support your own optimal food-mood connection.

Your Gut Microbiome Modulates Your Mood

As a refresher, the term *gut microbiome* refers to the ecosystem of bacteria, viruses, and fungi housed in our digestive system. There are about 100 trillion microbial cells in the human gut. Yes, I said *trillion*. That's ten times more than anywhere else in the human body.[5] And these microbial cells are constantly communicating with the brain.

Our gut bacteria "talk" to our brains by signaling our stress responses and even metabolizing our neurotransmitters (chemical messengers). Many researchers consider the enteric nervous system (the concentration of neurons in the gut) to be the second brain. As I mentioned previously, over 90 percent of serotonin is created in the gut. Our motivation chemical, dopamine, and calming chemical, GABA, get synthesized in the gut as well.[6]

Just as your very DNA and genetic blueprint are unique to you as an individual, so is the diversity of your microorganisms. Your early life exposure to stress and nutrition plays a role. Whether you were born vaginally or via C-section impacts microbial diversity. If you were breastfed, you received a greater diversity of species than if you were formula-fed. If you had a pet, lived on a farm or in a big city, played in the dirt or stayed inside all day—it all impacted the development of your microbiome. Did you receive frequent rounds of antibiotics or steroids as a child? Were you exposed to toxins or early life stressors? The bacterial species that developed in childhood as a result shaped your immune response, your stress response, and even your neurotransmitters.

The microorganisms in your body impact all aspects of health, which is why more research is being done on the impact of enhanced intestinal permeability (leaky gut) and many chronic disease states. Enhanced intestinal permeability happens when our exposure to stress, toxins, processed food, certain medications, and early-life microbial development leads to a breakdown in gut barrier function and causes bacterial imbalances (dysbiosis) of all kinds. This can create GI discomfort, food sensitivities, improper immune signaling, and, ultimately, inflammation.

Your gut microbes are so powerful that they regulate your stress response, normalize your cortisol levels, impact your cravings, and reduce inflammation. Some research studies suggest that probiotics (consumable microorganisms) improve mood to a similar degree as antianxiety and antidepressant medication.[7]

Here is where nutrition factors in. The health of your gut microbiome depends on the food you eat. Diversity of diet equals diversity of gut microbes, which is a good thing for mood support. In fact, the latest research suggests that diet is the most powerful aspect of creating a healthier microbiome. Eating a wide variety of fruits, vegetables, and fiber (such as nuts, seeds, whole grains, and beans) helps to feed those bacterial strains that do all the regulation for mood and health. On the flip side, the additives, pesticides, and processing of modern food do more harm than good to microbial diversity, causing overgrowths of opportunistic pathogens, creating more permeability to the gut lining, or leading to lack of microbial diversity.

I believe we'll be discussing the impact of the gut microbiome for many years to come because there is still so much we don't know. We do know that what the digestive system can digest, break down, absorb, and tolerate creates an ecosystem for health (or harm) to your mental well-being. But your mood isn't regulated by microbes alone. The content of what you eat—and how often—impacts your emotional well-being as well.

Your Blood Sugar Impacts Your Emotions

If you've ever felt "hangry," then you already know how a rapid drop in blood sugar can affect your mood. In that state, grabbing a snack flips the switch to calm again. What you might not realize, though, is how less dramatic changes in blood sugar can impact your emotions.

I'm a visual person, so when I'm describing how blood sugar impacts the body, I like to picture two types of roller coasters.

Because I live in Texas, I imagine them as two popular rides: the Texas Giant (big peaks and drops) and the Runaway Mine Train (smaller peaks and drops). When your body receives food, it must be broken down into glucose (sugar) to be released to the bloodstream and used for fuel. Glucose is your primary source of energy, but it needs to be supported by insulin, which acts as the roller coaster cart for the glucose. Insulin is released by the pancreas to get glucose into the cells. The size of the blood sugar roller coasters is impacted by the types of food we eat and how much glucose and insulin is released. So grab a fast pass, skip the line, and let's experience how the Texas Giant and the Runaway Mine Train illustrate different ways blood sugar can affect emotions.

The Texas Giant is the bigger roller coaster, and it demonstrates negative emotional outcomes. When a meal contains mostly refined carbohydrates (with very little protein, fat, or fiber), glucose and insulin can quickly spike upward, and then rapidly crash downward, which can feel pretty terrible. In fact, one research study showed that a married person felt more anger toward their spouse when they had low blood sugar levels.[8] Another study in teen boys showed that breakfasts higher in sugar dramatically spiked not just glucose and insulin, but the stress hormone adrenaline—up to five hours later![9] The symptoms experienced by the teen boys included sweating and shakiness. I imagine they may have felt like they were having a panic attack. Steeply falling glucose also triggers the release of cortisol, which, as you recall, is an important slower-acting stress hormone we need. But too much of a good thing like cortisol can lead to mood symptoms such as depression, anxiety, and even PTSD. When you're riding the Texas Giant, the rise and fall of blood sugar causes more than just hunger. It impacts your stress levels and emotions as well.

The Runaway Mine Train, with smaller peaks and shorter drops, is a gentler ride for the body. When you eat a more balanced meal consisting of complex carbohydrates (carbs that naturally contain more fiber, such as vegetables, legumes, and certain whole grains), fat, and protein, your insulin cart still prepares to take your glucose up and down, but not to the extremes the Texas Giant does. In fact, your mood stays more balanced, and you may even feel fuller for longer. No more hangry fights!

When the roller coaster ride gets too out of control, the body can grow resistant to the cart assistance of insulin. Insulin resistance happens when glucose keeps asking for a ride and insulin says, "Nah, man, I just did that!" This increases the likelihood of suffering a wide range of health complications. Perhaps most notable, insulin resistance *doubles* the risk of major depression,[10] confirming once again that blood sugar is connected to mood and mental health.

Your Nutrients Affect Your Nervous System

Receiving adequate nutrients helps your body feel safe from a nervous system perspective. When your body has what it needs from food, it can better regulate the stress response. It's important to have a balance of macronutrients (carbs, fat, and protein) to signal whole body safety, but it's also crucial to have enough micronutrients (vitamins and minerals). The amino acids (building blocks of protein) we get from protein, vitamins, and minerals are key ingredients to assembling neurotransmitters that make us feel good.

When I work with people on restorative nutrition, whether in a group program or one-on-one, the first thing we focus on is protein. Protein is the only macronutrient we don't store, and research suggests we use eight to ten grams of protein per hour. The body will store carbohydrates and fat, which is a beautiful, protective function! We crave carbs when we're depleted because we need quick energy via glucose, right? But without protein, we simply can't make the feel-good chemicals that lead our bodies to safety and calm.

The amino acids you break down from protein consumption help to form your neurotransmitters. You can't have serotonin without a tryptophan precursor, and you won't make dopamine without tyrosine. The head of medical education at Rupa Health, Dr. Kate Kresge, explains it this way:

> How do you make dopamine? There are two ingredients. Tyrosine and B6. You combine them, put them through an enzymatic reaction, and you have dopamine. That's it. If you aren't eating those nutrients in adequate amounts or absorbing them, you won't be able to make those neurohormones. Same thing with serotonin. You need tryptophan, B12, B9 (folate), and B6.[11]

In other words, just as you can't bake a tasty cake without all the ingredients, you won't build a healthy brain without all the ingredients to make feel-good neurotransmitters.

Imagine this scenario: You wake up after eight solid hours of sleep, but you're already late for work, so you rush to get ready. For a quick breakfast, you might make peanut butter toast to eat in the car, grab a breakfast bar on the way out the door, or pick up a muffin on the way to work. You will get anything from five to maybe ten grams of protein from these options, which may give you only an hour of sustained energy. At that point, you'll likely begin looking for some quick fuel, like my client Katie did when she snacked on Cheez-Its or got a fast-food value meal for lunch. However, if you start your day with twenty to thirty grams of protein, maybe with a few eggs scrambled with veggies, Greek yogurt with nuts and berries, or a quality protein shake, you will have more staying power for the rest of your day.

Researchers have studied the effects of low-protein diets on mice and found that mice on low-protein diets had negative behavior outcomes, such as poor cognition, hyperactivity, and agitation. When the mice were given amino acids, they reversed their symptoms.[12]

Other studies have shown that high-protein breakfasts boost dopamine levels.

While protein is the macronutrient I emphasize increasing first with my clients, I also prioritize micronutrients. Did you know that a recent study found twelve key nutrients to help the brain communicate with the body best? In 2018, the Antidepressant Food Score was created based on these nutrients: folate, iron, omega-3 fatty acids, magnesium, potassium, selenium, thiamine, vitamin A, vitamin B6, vitamin B12, vitamin C, and zinc. Researchers took these nutrients and created a list of foods that have the highest concentration of them. They ranked foods in percentages, giving them a food score. These foods include watercress (127 percent), spinach (97 percent), lettuces (74–99 percent), peppers (39–56 percent), cauliflower (41–42 percent), brussels sprouts (35 percent), lemons and strawberries (31 percent), and so many others.[13] That's great news for the fruit and veggie lover!

The bad news? According to psychiatrist Drew Ramsey, who helped create the Antidepressant Food Score list, "One-third of us are lacking zinc, 68 percent are deficient in magnesium, and a whopping 75 percent aren't getting enough folate."[14] Our bodies are designed to receive nutrients through food to thrive, but most of us would rather spend twenty minutes in the drive-through at rush hour than twenty minutes throwing together a stir-fry. In our hurried, fight-or-flight lifestyles, we often miss the importance of nutrients for neurotransmitter health. These brain nutrients are strong weapons in the battle against anxiety, depression, and other mental illnesses.

Making changes to your diet by supporting the gut microbiome, balancing blood sugar, and increasing nutrients is a powerful way to shift your mood and decrease physiological stress in your body. But like my client Katie, you may be wondering what the best approach is. Here comes the fun part!

Does Your Diet Lack Nutrients?

So many of the irritating symptoms we attribute to the natural process of aging are actually the ways our bodies communicate that they need more nutrients. See if you can relate to any of the following symptoms. Mark the ones you experience on a regular basis.

- ☐ I get dizzy or lightheaded if I don't eat frequently throughout the day.
- ☐ I crave sugar, carbs, and caffeine as pick-me-ups.
- ☐ I struggle with frequent colds, sinus infections, or viruses.
- ☐ I have skin issues such as rosacea, eczema, psoriasis, dermatitis, acne, or random rashes.
- ☐ I have muscle spasms or cramps.
- ☐ I suffer from joint pain.
- ☐ I feel bloated after meals and occasionally experience reflux.
- ☐ I have digestive issues such as gas, bloating, diarrhea, constipation, or all of these.
- ☐ I get numbness or tingling sensations in my hands and feet.
- ☐ I struggle with anxiety, depression, or poor focus.
- ☐ I have a hard time sleeping through the night.
- ☐ I experience a midafternoon energy slump.

Eating for Optimal Mental Health

I love the concept of *addition over restriction*. Yes, you are what you think about what you eat, your relationship with food as nourishment matters, and your approach to nutrients matters. So by adding in mindful eating practices along with key nutrients, you can optimize your mood and feel so much better—in mind *and* body.

I wish I'd learned these things much sooner than I did. Unfortunately, thanks to dieting, I never ate vegetables because I wanted to. For most of my life, I ate food that gave me the short-lived dopamine hits. (Remember the cherry pie story?) On the rare occasion that I dieted to lose weight, I relied on processed, low-calorie diet food, very little fruit (because "sugar"), and lots of green vegetables. Which meant I had salads with low-fat or sugar-free dressings. Hello, starvation mode, and goodbye, joy!

When I learned to eat for brain health and to improve my relationship with food as nourishment, I took a couple of years off from salads—not because I was restricting for dieting reasons but because salads made me think of hunger and diet plans. I wanted to enjoy eating vegetables, and forcing myself to eat iceberg lettuce with a couple of diced celery stalks and baby tomatoes topped with fat-free Italian dressing didn't help me learn to like them.

I chose *addition*. I loaded up on nutrient dense whole foods and experimented with roasting, sautéing, stir-frying, scrambling, and blending veggies into just about everything. In fact, all of the early recipes on my website were part of this discovery process and my mission to learn to throw things together from scratch. Do you know what I discovered? I've never met a veggie that doesn't get along with another one. I love roasting garlic cloves, broccoli, onions, and sweet potatoes together. I use frozen vegetables, and I blend frozen riced cauliflower into smoothies when I'm in a rush. I'll top anything with peppery arugula, and I've determined that roasted bell peppers taste like candy.

When I combined a healthier food relationship with good-mood foods, I never felt deprived or tempted to diet via restriction again. That doesn't mean I didn't practice restraint in some areas. However, as I learned what foods made me feel good, it was easier to say goodbye to those that didn't. I simply no longer felt hooked on the nutrient-depleted, ultra-processed foods.

And that's exactly what I worked on with Katie, who felt overwhelmed by nutrition advice, didn't know how to step away from the Cheez-Its, and desired consistency. By learning to manage her stress, increasing her protein content, and shifting her diet to a wide variety of whole food sources that she enjoyed and that kept her full, she felt better. When she felt better, she felt less driven by cravings for the processed foods that didn't give her lasting energy.

If making changes like these still feels like an overwhelming hurdle for you, that's okay. I completely understand. Food brings up so many emotions, and change can be scary. But keep in mind that it's difficult to heal when the food you're eating for comfort or safety is keeping you in a physiological state of stress. If the food you're frequently consuming contains refined carbs and sugars that quickly spike and then drop your blood sugar, it will send a stress alert to your entire body. If it's ultra-processed, containing artificial chemicals that are difficult to break down, the process of breaking it down will create stress for your digestive system.

No matter how you choose to support your mind-body connection with food, remember that your choices aren't *morality* issues. What you eat isn't going to make or break your relationship with God, others, or even yourself. But the nutrients you consume directly impact the way you feel, and the way you feel impacts how you show up to live out your purpose. On the other hand, it's also important to remember that your choices with food aren't *virtue* issues either—they don't make you a better or more holy person. The apostle Paul reminds us, "Food will not commend us to God. We are no worse off if we do not eat, and no better off if we do" (1 Corinthians 8:8). Whether you are gluten-free, dairy-free, or sugar-free, what you choose to eat doesn't determine your status as a believer.

You don't have to live enslaved to food rules that restrict you and keep you miserable. You don't have to be held hostage by your next candy craving. You don't have to bow to the idols of diet, wellness, or processed food culture. However, what you choose to eat will impact your nervous system and your mental health. When you feel better—mentally and physically—you serve better.

The Great Gluten Debate

Gluten is a protein found in all wheat products, and there is a great deal of evidence-based research about its potential negative impact on mental health, especially for those with illnesses such as schizophrenia and bipolar disorder.[15] Gluten consumption releases a protein called zonulin, which increases enhanced intestinal permeability for everyone, regardless of sensitivity, allergy, or Celiac diagnosis.[16] This can lead to chronic inflammation. The presence of the commonly used pesticide glyphosate further affects the gut barrier function, leading to nutrient deficiencies.[17]

Here's another fact many don't know: When gluten is ingested, it breaks down into a compound called gluteomorphin. Did you catch the word *morphine* in there? Turns out, one potential reason bread products make us feel so good is because they're literally acting on our opioid receptors. While gluten can break down into gluteomorphin, dairy breaks down into casomorphin. Some people are more sensitive to this calming effect of dairy and wheat than others, which may be why you find yourself drawn to comfort substances such as Cheez-Its.

My prayer for you is the same as Paul's prayer for the Thessalonian church two millennia ago: "May God himself, the God who makes everything holy and whole, make you holy and whole, put you together—spirit, soul, and body—and keep you fit for the coming of our Master, Jesus Christ" (1 Thessalonians 5:23, MSG).

MAKING THE MIND-BODY CONNECTION

Here are two things you can do to optimize healthy brain function through nutrition. Keep in mind that this isn't a diet; it's a way to incorporate brain food via small steps, tuning in to how your brain and body respond in the process.

- ***Practice addition over restriction.*** For one week, focus on adding the following into your meals:

  > *Twenty to thirty grams of protein at each meal.* Aim for 100 grams total by the end of each day.

  > *Five different vegetables each day.* I like to play the color game here. Include a red, green, orange, purple, and yellow/white plant food every day. Make it fun!

  > *Two or three different fresh fruits each day.* Play the color game here, too! Switch it up so you don't get bored.

Throughout the week, focus on how you're feeling. How does it feel to eat that much protein or produce? What cravings do you have, if any? Are there any changes in your energy levels or sleep patterns? What has shifted for you?

- ***Practice restraint.*** After practicing addition, devote the next week to focusing on restraint. Instead of complete restriction, which feels negative, cultivate curiosity about the foods you eat out of habit that may not be offering much energy or mental health support. What foods do you turn to in stress or heightened emotional unease? If you feel comfortable doing so, practice restraint by refraining from eating on autopilot. Focus on eating only the foods that allow you to stay present in your body. If numbing out on a box of Cheez-Its or other snack foods is a trap for you, get curious about the habit and practice a period of restraint to tune in to why that might be so. Is it the food itself or the way you feel when you eat the food? There will also be a place for fun foods (don't even try to suggest I stop eating at my favorite Mexican food restaurant), but if it's a habit that's distressing for you and interfering with your ability to incorporate nutrient-dense options, restraint might be a good option to consider.

12

WEIGHT ISSUES AND RESTORING BODY PEACE

"I'm not blonde, and I'm not skinny. Therefore, I'm not attractive." I wrote this in a journal I kept during my senior year of high school. I'd embarked on a mission to weigh a specific number through a particular diet. Thanks to my new friend Zoloft (the antidepressant I was prescribed for my persistent depression), I gained twenty-five pounds between the end of my sophomore year and the beginning of my senior year. As a result, I spent a lot of time isolating, reading historical romances, and writing fictional stories. I felt that my weight was holding me back from enjoying my senior year, and only through weight loss would I feel like myself again.

I believed the diet would give me a new life. A new identity. A new way to really love the skin I was in—because it would come in a much smaller body. According to my journal, I was drinking two special protein drinks a day and cutting out all carbs, sugar, and caffeine. I was supposedly "retraining my body" to digest and store food, and there was an 85 percent chance I would "NEVER" gain my weight back.

Listen, I've struggled with body image since I was eight years old, but this diet had me obsessed. I wrote a lot about what I couldn't have and the food I dreamed of, but also how the restrictions were "worth it." According to later entries, I almost passed out at swim team practice because I was so calorie deprived. However, as the weight began to fall off, I grew more confident. I stopped isolating and started going out more. I developed an interest in not one, not two, but three different boys at my school, and I was proud of all the attention I received from my newly improved, smaller body. I couldn't wait to get a belly button ring when my waist measured a specific number.

But I never hit my goal weight. My body halted five pounds away. During the summer after I graduated, the weight started to creep back on as I left starvation mode and my metabolism rebalanced. It depressed me. I was a failure. My body was a failure. Nobody would want to be around me at my higher weight. Eventually, my journal entries turned more manic, a reflection of what was happening at the brain level. By the end of the summer, I was experiencing symptoms of mania, including risky behavior, grandiosity, lack of sleep, and increased goal-directed activity. And then my immune system crashed. I was diagnosed with mononucleosis and bipolar disorder within weeks of each other.

Yo-yo dieting was a disaster for my mental and physical health, and I hear similar stories from many women in my office. To be clear, there were many factors that played a role in my diagnoses, so I don't completely blame the restrictive diet. I had tried other diets before, though none as extreme or with such dramatic results. It's hard not to wonder if the dieting flipped a switch in my nervous system that heightened my body's psychoneuroimmunological response and played at least some role in my mental health condition.

Throughout adolescence and early adulthood, I sought out many solutions to perfect my body. However, chasing the next miracle diet only put me at war with my body and its needs. It led me to place most of my trust in a magical plan, but very little trust in my own body's ability to find balance. It wasn't until years later when I learned to create acceptance for my body and restore body peace that I began to heal.

Many of my clients list weight loss as a goal and express dissatisfaction with their size or number on the scale. Others suffer from mysterious weight loss that stumps them and their medical practitioners, leading them to feel dissatisfied and frustrated with their bodies as well. I have to clarify for my clients that while I am concerned about their nutrition, I am not a diet coach. In fact, I don't typically accept clients whose only goal is intentional weight loss. That's because dieting for intentional weight loss inevitably fails, with 95 percent of dieters regaining the weight within two years.[1]

A huge aspect of the healing journey is creating safety in the body you have, not pining for the body you want to have. It's a cultural belief that having the ideal body is the key to unlocking body peace. But take it from me—mastering a goal weight doesn't lead to mastering internal satisfaction. In fact, the quest for the perfect number on a scale can often lead to more distress. Dissatisfaction in your body and chasing the magical number creates a perpetual lack of body peace. I define body peace as acceptance that your body is always on your side, working to alert you to symptoms. Sometimes those symptoms are pleasant and sometimes they are not. Instead of promoting dieting to clients, I focus on helping them create body peace by restoring what the

Should You Pursue Intentional Weight Loss?

Everyone has a set-point weight that makes their body feel best, so if you feel like that number has crept up to one that doesn't feel right for you, I believe you. I know it can cause discomfort. However, here's why I don't recommend trying extreme caloric restriction: Your body is always looking for balance, so by nature, it resists sustained weight loss by dropping the basal metabolic rate every time you drastically drop your calorie consumption for an extended period. One example of this was documented by *The Biggest Loser* contestants in a study that showed "people who have lost large amounts of weight must adhere to an extremely low-calorie intake in order to maintain that weight loss."[2]

If you are struggling with weight, a crash diet might work against you in the long-term. To make sustainable changes, focus on health-promoting behaviors such as decreasing refined carbs and sugars and increasing whole food sources of nutrition. Your body breaks down calories from whole foods very differently than calories from processed foods, and they lead to a natural stopping point; whereas processed foods are designed to be overconsumed. Create small, sustainable goals over time, such as eliminating sweetened drinks first (they lead only to more hunger and cravings anyway), increasing water intake, or choosing to cook most of your whole-food meals instead of grabbing fast food or takeout. These small changes should be ones you can maintain for a lifetime, not short-term. For example, I haven't had a soda in over a decade and have zero desire for one. It doesn't improve my life, so I'm fine exercising restraint. However, I occasionally indulge in gluten-free baked goods, and I pay close attention to how I feel when I have them. Foods with MSG and other artificial additives cause me to overconsume, so if I sense an overwhelming desire for more without feeling satisfied, I reevaluate whether that treat is worth it.

When you make changes with sustainable change in mind, instead of a diet plan for only a few months, you're more likely to stick with it—and weight loss will be a side effect of a body in balance, instead of a body being punished.

body needs to feel balanced. But before we can get there, we must understand that weight issues are *symptoms of other underlying imbalances*, not causes.

Understanding the Reasons Behind Weight Struggles

Quick fixes for weight loss don't fix the root cause of the issue. You can still struggle with health issues even with an optimal body mass index (BMI) number—in fact, that's a reason many chronic health issues get overlooked for those in a smaller body. Because weight changes are symptoms of other underlying issues, I like to ask the question, "Why is the body choosing to store weight right now?" The answer is usually not as simple as "calories in, calories out" or a lack of willpower and discipline.

I want to shift the way you view weight issues because there are many valid reasons the body might struggle to maintain a consistent weight. Medication can bring about weight gain as a side effect, and even the effects of chronic stress, toxin exposure, and shifting hormones will skew the number on the scale up or down. While there are numerous underlying root causes for weight fluctuations, four of the most common—and most overlooked—include side effects from medication, physiological stressors, toxicity, and hormonal changes.

Side effects from medication. One vastly overlooked cause of weight struggles is prescription medications. One example is antidepressants, also known as selective serotonin reuptake inhibitors (SSRIs). Some studies indicate that SSRIs cause weight gain due to the potential disruption of strains of bacteria that regulate body weight, such as lactobacillus.[3] Other studies suggest weight gain from SSRIs is an effect of an increased appetite and craving for carbohydrates.[4] One researcher affirms, "It has long been known that antipsychotic medications can affect weight, diabetes, and metabolism."[5] There are many other medications (prescription and over-the-counter) that have been documented to alter weight, including oral contraceptives, steroids, beta blockers, and antihistamines. Even when we understand that weight gain is a side effect, the inner battle remains, leading many to wonder, "Do I have to sacrifice fitting into my favorite jeans to feel relief from these unpleasant symptoms?"

Physiological stressors. Rapid weight gain or loss can be a sign of an internal imbalance. This imbalance might be caused by physiological stressors such as chronic inflammation. Blood sugar fluctuations impact insulin signaling, lead to weight issues, and create poor signaling of hunger and fullness cues. Overconsumption of nutrient-poor processed food is a stressor for the body that creates a vicious cycle, leading it to seek out more hyperpalatable foods that increase weight storage and decrease the nutrients needed to activate metabolic processes to lose weight. Gut microbial imbalances can lead to increased hunger and weight storage. Grief, trauma, or stress can increase physiological distress, leading to weight changes.[6] For some, food intolerances increase physiological stress, which can absolutely lead to weight changes.[7]

Toxicity. Even our fat cells can contribute to our weight struggles, because fat cells are extremely protective. Adipose tissue (body fat) is a handy storage tank for toxins. When the body struggles to detoxify from environmental chemicals and there aren't enough nutrients and antioxidants to transform and excrete the toxins, fatty tissue holds on to it. Consistently overeating food that is devoid of nutrients and poorly absorbed is a good way to guarantee toxic storage as well.[8] I call this being "overfed and undernourished." It's not just the caloric content of the food that's the problem; it's the lack of nutrients in high-calorie processed foods that keep the body starved and consistently hungry. When much of our frequently consumed foods are designed to make us crave them, it's difficult to tap into our ghrelin and leptin hormones (that tell us to start and stop eating),[9] so the storage cycle perpetuates.

Hormonal changes. Any imbalance in reproductive hormones can create weight struggles, but one lesser-discussed cause of sudden weight change occurs during reproductive hormone decline for women over thirty-five. During this perimenopause period, ovaries gradually cease production of estrogen, progesterone, and testosterone and leave it up to two other production factories in the body: the adrenal glands and adipose tissue. Chronic stress can decrease the adrenal glands' ability to support reproductive hormones, so if you've been running on autopilot your whole life, it leaves adipose tissue to support hormone production, causing the body to store more fat. Once again, this is an incredibly protective design from our Creator, but it sure doesn't feel helpful when you're eating the same things you always have and suddenly can't button your shorts.

If weight is an ongoing struggle for you, I want you to know I see you. I know weight is a sensitive topic. Perhaps you've been told to just "eat less and exercise more," and you feel shame because of where you landed on the BMI chart. Maybe you were told you're "fine" because your BMI is normal or below normal, but you feel anything but fine. Perhaps a well-meaning physician made stinging remarks, or a trainer pushed you for weight loss or gain. Or it's possible your friends or family members make weight-related comments, which trigger feelings of embarrassment and helplessness. I've experienced all the above, and I know how much it hurts.

No matter what the reason your body has chosen to store weight, I hope you can see that there's often a reason your body holds on to extra weight. Your body is on your side, even when it shows up differently than you'd like. Understanding the root dynamics is a stepping stone to finding body peace. But there's one more obstacle that often interferes with body peace. And that has to do with different types of noise that threaten your body peace.

Noise That Disrupts Body Peace

The way food and body image are addressed in the culture at large often causes major disruptions in how we feel about our bodies, creating excess mental noise that makes it difficult for us to listen to our intuitive needs for nourishment. Thanks to messaging that weight gain is a result of laziness and lack of motivation or discipline, many women feel shame for their weight gain. They blame themselves, firing up the critic within. On the flip side, there are also many women who lose weight without intending to. They, too, endure judgment from others and themselves. This constant stream of noise primes you for body punishment rather than body partnership and is a threat to sustained body peace. There are four main types of disruptive noise you may encounter when it comes to your relationship with food: diet noise, food noise, nutrition noise, and your own noise.

Diet noise. If you've tried even one diet in your lifetime, you know that even when you finish the diet, the internal noise remains. Whether you counted points or calories, macros or carbs, you likely created a narrative in your head surrounding your eating habits. Unfortunately, relying only on numbers can separate you from your own intuitive needs and create mistrust in your body. I used to mentally tally up calories throughout my day, to the point where it was a distraction from enjoying the food itself. It brought excess stress to my brain that took me away from trusting the needs of my own body based on my own hunger and fullness cues. As psychologist and "Health at Every Size" advocate Dr. Linda Bacon writes, "Failed attempts at losing weight make people feel like failures, and even those who succeed feel a never-ending pressure to retain that success that will always limit their ability to feel comfortable around food and in their bodies."[10]

Food noise. The language you use for the food you eat—such as placing food into categories of "good" and "bad"—can be negative for your relationship with your body. For example, my client Kaya was so consumed with food guilt after indulging in a food she considered "bad" or unhealthy that it created digestive distress. Another client, Tamara, was so terrified of salt that she said even the thought of added sodium in food made her ankles and feet swell in response. She was afraid to flavor her food with salt because she didn't trust her body's ability to use it.

Nutrition noise. The overabundance of nutrition information, much of it conflicting, can disrupt body peace. A woman who heard me speak at an event approached me afterward and said, "Thanks to you, I let myself eat bananas again!" She had been avoiding bananas due to what she heard about their high glycemic content. I was thrilled to hear that she was enjoying bananas again. (By the way, if I'm remembered as the health coach who tells you it's okay to eat a banana, then my work here is done.) Nobody should feel guilty for eating a food God created in nature to nourish us and give us energy. Yet, thanks to nutrition information overload and years of being told what not to eat, we restrict things like bananas. We'd rather choose a diet-brand processed bar made of synthetic ingredients than something that has been nourishing people for thousands of years.

Your own noise. The language you use to talk to *yourself* about food can prevent you from activating the parasympathetic (rest-and-digest) state. Your fear of food and worry about what it will do to your body can send a threat signal to your brain, which in turn causes your hypothalamus to release corticotropin-releasing factor (CRF) to every organ and cell in your body to activate stress mode. This disrupts digestion by causing the gut to contract more, sometimes resulting in diarrhea. The stomach can slow down and reverse to send contents upward, resulting in indigestion. The gut wall will become more permeable, and increased blood flow through the lining of the stomach and intestines can cause undigested food particles to elicit an immune response, creating food sensitivities. The entire process brings anything but peace to your body.

Even your internal dialogue of "shoulds" can interfere with body peace. *I should be eating more vegetables. I should stop drinking soda. I shouldn't be gaining this weight. I should be seeing more results by now.* May I make a suggestion? Stop shoulding all over yourself! Be gentle with yourself and how you talk about food and your body.

So many of my clients feel the weight of what they should or shouldn't be eating for their health, and it often results in a religiosity that's harmful. For many Christians coming out of a "purity culture" mindset, restrictive eating is another way to feel pure and holy. An obsession with clean eating is on the rise as more information about the toxic chemicals and additives in our foods becomes increasingly available. With the advent of programs such as Whole30 and the Daniel Fast, it is appealing to want to go back to nature, to the way God intended food, and take an extreme stance on the evils of processed food.

But for many, such a fastidious approach to food only creates a new obsession with weight. It can even cause division, as health enthusiasts can be seen as pious Pharisees who are judging others on their consumption of Doritos. Wellness culture can start to look a lot like diet culture. But then anti-diet culture can appear to shame anyone who wants to try to stop consuming Doritos because they don't like how they feel when they eat them. The messages we get from all sides leave us feeling like we're living in a state of constant contradiction.

The primary problem with all the noise is that we end up looking for quick fixes and cure-alls without reflecting on what we need as individuals. This is why diets are so appealing at first. *If I can just do one thing for a short amount of time, lose the weight, and*

Phrases That Disrupt Body Peace

Remove these common phrases from your vocabulary to pursue body peace.

Cheat meal. This implies you are being deceptive/sneaky with your body. You don't have to be deceptive when you are on the same team!

It's not on my plan; I can't. A statement like this puts ownership of what you choose to eat into someone else's hands. But remember, you get to choose what's best for you. You also can choose to say no for yourself rather than because of what the plan says. Saying, "I don't want to eat that right now," allows you to advocate for yourself and take ownership of your needs.

Guilt-free dessert. Choosing to eat dessert and find pleasure in food is not a moral failing, so all desserts, by design, should be guilt-free. We were not given fruit and honey to deprive ourselves of sweetness. The caution is to avoid using sweets and other foods to numb emotional pain. Using any food or other substance to numb pain can result in significant emotional and physical consequences.

Good food/bad food. Different types of food perform different functions in your body and are received differently. Some food makes you feel better than other food. But that doesn't make eating any food an issue of morality; nor does it make you a good or bad person.

I already blew it today. This is a sweeping judgment based on one food choice, at one point in the day. The negativity itself can alter digestion and bring distress throughout the body, which creates unnecessary stress, leading to more regrettable food decisions.

---

then hit my goal, I can go back to life as usual. But that isn't body partnership; it's body punishment.

It's time to partner with and befriend your body through the words you use and consume as well as through the foods you eat. And I promise, it's not as difficult as you might think. When you partner with your body to create a safe environment, body peace follows.

Creating an Environment for Peace

Your body needs to feel safe to heal, but with so many underlying root causes and internal noises holding you back, it may feel more like you're playing Sisyphus with your progress. Before you push forward with a weight loss plan, may I ask you to consider that the weight you really need to lose might have nothing to do with fat cells? What if the weight you need to rid your body of is the weight of chronic stress—the emotional and physiological kind? What if truly being healthy isn't an issue of food input but one of mental input?

If you struggle with added weight and you believe that extra weight is harmful to your health, then healing *is* a necessary step in the process. But healing will not come from creating more stress on a new diet. Healing happens when your body feels nourished—externally and internally. Body peace starts with the basics, the things that bring balance to all bodies of all shapes and sizes: primary nourishment and secondary nourishment.

Primary nourishment. Your body must be out of fight, flight, freeze, or fawn to experience peace. This requires receiving your primary source of nourishment from God, your relationships with others, and your own sense of purpose. Experiencing joy and gratitude are powerful messengers that send signals of peace throughout the body. Awe is a powerful emotion that can reduce the presence of inflammatory cytokines in the body.[11] Your body receives boosts of oxytocin (a neurotransmitter that helps you to feel connected and happy) from being with people you love and doing things you love to do. When you partner with your body in gentleness and self-compassion, with awe for how God designed it, it can restore peace.

Secondary nourishment. To create an environment of peace, your body needs nutrients from food. It needs sufficient protein to break down into amino acids, which are needed to create neurotransmitters. It needs B vitamins and magnesium to help you manage stress. It needs fiber-rich vegetables, nuts, and grains to create short-chain fatty acids to feed your brain positive signals. It needs mitochondria in your cells functioning optimally with these nutrients to provide your body with ATP for energy. It needs to be able to create beneficial bacteria to form neurotransmitters that keep you calm, happy, and motivated. This won't happen by restricting food. This will happen when you receive *enough* food that is nutrient-dense, and when you partner with your body to mindfully engage in consuming food.

Here's a loving challenge: Consider how you might create an environment of peace in your body through primary and secondary nourishment. You can't expect your body—or brain—to function optimally when you aren't creating space for safety and peace. As author Christine Valters Paintner so beautifully shares, "I am convinced that learning to live in our bodies, to truly embrace both the profound dignity and pleasure as well as the tenderness and sometimes excruciating vulnerability of them, is the most important work we can do."[12]

You were created for wholeness and purpose. You were given one body as the active vessel to live that purpose. And guess what? You are just the right you-size for the God-sized mission in front of you.

MAKING THE MIND-BODY CONNECTION

The purpose of the following exercises is to choose partnership with your body and view it as a friend. Increasing appreciation for your body may feel weird or self-indulgent, but it's a helpful way to tune in to your body's needs and see it as an ally instead of an adversary.

LIVE BEYOND YOUR LABEL

- ***Write a letter to your body.*** Address your body directly and express how you feel about it. For example, you might express appreciation for how your body has protected you and kept you safe, even when you didn't feel safe. You might need to ask for forgiveness for times you ignored your body's needs or sought to punish it through food restriction, intense exercise, or negative self-talk. You might reflect on when the battle with your body started and what core beliefs arose from it. Then ask your body what it needs from you going forward. Close the letter expressing your commitment to paying more attention to your body and partnering with it for healing. If writing your own letter feels too difficult for you right now, that's okay. The next activity may be more comfortable for you.

- ***Read this letter to your body out loud.*** Find a quiet space where you won't be distracted and can read the following letter aloud. Take a few deep breaths before and after getting started, paying attention to the sensations your body sends you as you read.

Dear Body,

I know we've been disconnected for a long time. I've tried many ways to find contentment with you, and they all have left me more frustrated. I want to start again—to create safety and nourishment for you today and every day. I want to partner with you in nourishment and peace instead of punishment and discontentment. I apologize for shutting you out for such a long time. I understand that nothing about your design is an accident. You're a masterpiece created by God to be a vessel for his Spirit, and to enable me to live out my purpose in the world. I know my Creator cares about my body, which means I can care about you too. I commit to honoring you with intention going forward.

Love,
Me

PART 4

LEARN to address stress
IDENTIFY the root issues
add VARIETY to your diet

EXERCISE YOUR BODY AND BRAIN

Author and business advisor Darren Hardy explores what he calls the "Compound Effect," which is the way small daily actions compound over time to create big changes. He writes, "The most challenging aspect of the Compound Effect is that we have to keep working away for a while, consistently and efficiently, before we begin to see the payoff."[1] In the same way, the tiniest spark can lead to the biggest blaze, which is the idea behind my company and podcast name, Sparking Wholeness. Sometimes it's the little things, the ones that seem the most basic or unnoticeable, that catalyze the most profound transformations. But those little things must be practiced consistently.

Part 4 focuses on the fourth step of learning to live beyond your label, which is exercising your body and brain through the way you live out your days, weeks, months, and so on. Your daily practices of engaging your brain and body matter. Your resilience is impacted by your ability to regulate your emotions, move your body to engage your brain, and make space for healing rest. These small steps, compounded by the other tools you've learned, are the sparks that can ignite a blaze of wholeness in your life.

13

ENGAGING IN HEALTHY EMOTIONAL REGULATION

Have you ever woken up in a great mood, ready to take on the day, but then you were disrupted by one seemingly tiny event? Maybe your car is running low on gas, so you have to refuel on the way to work, which makes you late. Or you're halfway to your child's school when she realizes she forgot her lunch, so you need to turn around, making *her* late. Or maybe you're in the middle of an important task and you realize you forgot to respond to a time-sensitive email, so you have to switch tasks, respond, then switch back. From that moment on, the rest of your day feels out of sync, like you're playing catch-up all day.

Sometimes all it takes is one small interaction with another person to throw you off. Perhaps you receive a cryptic email from your boss with an invitation to his office but no context of why (so you spend the rest of the day until the meeting thinking you're in trouble). Or you receive a text message from a friend in crisis, and while you want to be a caring friend, you know that engaging will deplete your energy.

For some, these scenarios may be minor inconveniences, but for others, they're trip wires for the inner critic to start shouting accusations. At least, that's how it is for me. Nothing disrupts my inner peace more than getting thrown off by the unexpected and not being able to regain my footing. However, as I've grown in self-awareness and learned to practice healthy emotional regulation, I can more quickly regain perspective and a strong dose of peace.

Emotional regulation is the ability to recognize, understand, and manage your emotions in response to the world around you. When you're emotionally regulated, you can better experience the effects of pleasant emotions and limit the impact of unpleasant emotions so they aren't as draining. Healthy emotional regulation involves being aware of what triggers you and finding what you need to feel safe and regulated again.

Because each person's capacity for stress is different, we also have a varying capacity for regulating our emotions in response to the intensity of our external environment. To advocate for our own health and well-being, we need to be aware of our need for healthy emotional regulation—and that starts with recharging our emotional batteries.

Your Emotional Batteries Need to Be Recharged

Your emotional batteries have a capacity limit, and they can run low more or less frequently depending on how well you practice emotional regulation. The goal of healthy emotional regulation is to have the flexibility to adapt from a felt sense of discomfort right back to a felt sense of safety. This isn't a decision our bodies can make for us, so we have to practice various forms of regulation to improve our adaptability.

ENGAGING IN HEALTHY EMOTIONAL REGULATION

We're going to focus on three forms of emotional regulation: self-regulation, co-regulation, and soul regulation. Each of these comes from our primary nourishment—our relationships with ourselves, others, and God. All three forms of regulation bring safety, and each creates its own positive ripple effect on the body and mind.

Self-Regulation Creates Peace

Self-regulation enables us to access our own self-soothing tools for support. It helps us to control impulses and avoid getting derailed by minor interruptions in the flow of our day. As simple as it sounds, too many of us struggle with this because we weren't taught healthy self-regulation tools growing up. For example, you might have been taught or picked up the message that it isn't safe to express frustration or sadness. Or maybe you were taught that complaining is a sin, so you swallowed your disappointment. If you grew up feeling like you had to suppress or deny certain emotions, your ability to learn how to safely regulate those emotions was interrupted. So even when something small happens that changes your plans or expectations, you don't know what to do with the emotion it evokes. This leaves you feeling *dys*regulated.

Here's an example: My client Riley experienced a shocking revelation in middle school when she learned that the man she considered her dad was not her biological father. Now, anytime she receives new information without warning, it scares her. One day, her boss called her into a meeting without any heads-up on what the meeting was about. This panicked Riley. *Am I getting fired? What did I do wrong? Is he demoting me?* As it turned out, he simply valued her opinion and wanted her input on the topic at hand.

Healthy self-regulation enables you to assess the real-time threat level of the dysregulating incident with confidence. Having confidence that you can tackle any interruption in your day brings peace. It lessens the fear of "what if" and keeps you grounded in the "right now."

Trauma researcher Bessel van der Kolk writes, "Self-regulation depends on having a friendly relationship with your body."[1] To experience healthy self-regulation, you must tune in to the needs of your body and listen to the signals it gives you. In Riley's situation, she knew that the sensations her body was sending her were those of fear and overwhelm. She recognized that even though she had no logical need to panic, her body did the panicking for her in anticipation of a perceived threat. Because she recognized this alert, she was able to ground herself, practicing some deep breaths before entering the meeting.

As you've learned, because of the incredible design of the human brain, your body is fighting for you, looking for balance. Often the body communicates through sensations such as what Riley experienced. Self-regulation brings balance back to your body and creates peace.

Co-Regulation Creates Connection

Co-regulation is like self-regulation, but instead of working to calm yourself, you are being supported emotionally by someone else who is in a calm, regulated state. It occurs when two or more people work together to manage emotions and responses to stress or discomfort. For example, you may have experienced co-regulation when you received comfort from a friend during a difficult life season or when you comforted someone else. This brings relational connection and allows each person to feel validated, seen, and heard for who they are and in what they're experiencing. And when you already have tools for self-regulation, it creates stronger awareness of others' needs for co-regulation as well. Your sense of peace can bring comfort to them, enabling them to feel connected despite feelings of emotional dysregulation.

ENGAGING IN HEALTHY EMOTIONAL REGULATION

Co-regulation is not the same as codependency. Codependency is an unhealthy relational dynamic in which one person is excessively dependent on the other, and the person being depended on derives their identity from or feels a sense of pride in being needed. This leads the supportive person to offer continuous aid to feel validated. However, their support keeps the dependent person dependent rather than helping them to grow, change, or take personal responsibility for their circumstances and choices. This is why it's termed *co*dependency—because both people are dependent on one another in unhealthy ways. The relational imbalance decreases independence and ability to self-regulate, because both people are solely relying on the other to regulate for them. This can lead both to disconnect from their own needs and leave them too dependent on the other.

In healthy co-regulation, both people receive security and comfort from one another as needed, without depleting the supportive person's energy. This leads to connection and greater personal awareness. Co-regulation might occur one-on-one, such as during a deep discussion with a trusted friend, or it can occur in a large group setting, such as during a worship service in which people stand together as they sing and express gratitude. Maintaining eye contact, taking a walk, or engaging in nonsexual touch (such as a warm hug) are also tools for co-regulation. Co-regulation is why therapy is so powerful. When you share your story with a safe person who receives it with kindness and compassion, you feel more connected not just to your personal experience but to the other person as well.

Let's go back to the example I shared about Riley and her boss. Because the request caused her to be fearful, she texted a friend: "Hey, I just got a weird email from my boss, asking to meet with me. I feel nervous, but I'm not sure if I have reason to be. I don't have time to talk, but can you pray for me?" Her friend immediately responded, "On it. I'm praying for your peace of mind and for strength in the meeting." Receiving that text from her friend, as simple as it was, helped to take the intensity of Riley's emotions down a few notches. She felt seen and connected to another human, and that created more regulation.

Soul-Regulation Creates Hope

While self-regulation turns your focus inside of you and co-regulation turns your focus outside of you, soul-regulation turns your focus upward—to the God who created all your emotions. Soul-regulation is finding hope in your purpose by choosing to stay connected to God. When your emotional battery is plugged into your Creator, receiving sustenance from him, you gain a renewed sense of purpose, which brings hope. And get this—there's research demonstrating that a greater sense of purpose is linked to better health outcomes.[2] Every part of you benefits from soul-regulation.

Jesus referred to this type of soul connection when he encouraged his followers to, "*Abide* in me, and I in you. As the branch cannot bear fruit by itself, unless it *abides* in the vine, neither can you, unless you *abide* in me" (John 15:4, emphasis added). The Greek word translated "abide" is *meno*. It means "to remain, live, dwell; to be in a state that begins and continues."[3] And Jesus' metaphor of a vine and a branch perfectly captures the kind of relationship God wants to have with us—one of continuous connection.

When we neglect our connection with God, we're like a branch that's partially or wholly disconnected from its nutrient source. As soon as life throws a few storms our way, we'll struggle to bounce back and live out our God-given purpose, much as a branch would be unable to fulfill its purpose of bearing fruit. You and I are born with a longing for purpose. When we choose to engage with God on an ongoing basis—to abide in him—we not only remain connected to our primary nourishment but also are reminded that we are part of something bigger than us, that we have a purpose because we belong to and are beloved by God.

When Riley received the fear-inducing message from her boss, she understood her need for self-regulation as well as co-regulation. But as Riley's brain was spinning from the notification on her computer screen, she looked to her keyboard, where she had written a verse on a sticky note weeks prior: "For the LORD will be your confidence and will keep your foot from being caught" (Proverbs 3:26). That reminder—that God is her confidence—gave her another way to help regulate the surge of emotion she experienced.

Remaining connected to our spiritual sustenance also brings us the hope and nourishment we need when we're derailed and drained by life's curveballs. This isn't to say that closing our eyes and thinking about our God-given purpose is going to take away all our frustration. It won't. The demands of life are constant, and many times we react instinctively before we can respond intentionally. But I do know this: During times of irritation and struggle, when I check in with myself and evaluate what deficiency of primary nourishment is the biggest, I usually find that what I need most is soul-regulation—to connect with God. For me, that's often the missing puzzle piece to bring me hope. Maybe it is for you too.

All forms of healthy emotional regulation—whether self-regulation, co-regulation, or soul-regulation—require awareness of the life glitches that throw us off. That's why it's crucial to understand our triggers and how they impact us.

Understanding Your Triggers

Triggered is a term that gets thrown around a lot these days. Whether you believe the phrase is overused or not, the fact remains that everyone gets triggered. Triggers are alerts based on memories of unpleasant or traumatic events, and their purpose is to notify us of impending danger.

The first thing to understand about triggers is that they exist to protect us. Every time we experience a stressor or a perceived threat, that information hits a portion of our brains in the limbic system called the amygdala. The amygdala is God's gift for our survival. It is responsible for the way we startle when someone tries to scare us, and it activates automatically, without any conscious effort on our part.

Due to chronic stress, trauma, neurotransmitter imbalances, or brain injury, you might find yourself with an overactive amygdala. If you've ever experienced a panic attack, you know what it feels like. The panic arrives without warning, and your body has a physiological response to what is most often an imagined rather than actual threat.

This is where the developed prefrontal cortex comes into play. If you are over the age of twenty-five, you likely have a fully developed prefrontal cortex. If you recall from chapter 3, it's the adult portion of our brains that causes us to stop and say, "Wait a minute. This event/circumstance/person is not really anything to panic about. I'm going to be okay." Our prefrontal cortex helps us to make clear, rational choices, and it keeps us from impulsivity.

The other important thing to understand about triggers is that it's physiologically impossible to access the prefrontal cortex and recognize a trigger as a practice alert, not a present threat, when you are in a state of chronic stress. For example, when you're overworked and burned out, living off reheated coffee and another last-minute drive-through order, stress magnifies your awareness of triggers and intensifies their detrimental effect on your well-being. In fact, when you're running around dysregulated, driven by your triggers, you might react impulsively and be tempted to do things you'll later regret. It's like Paul says, "For I have the desire to do what is right, but not the ability to carry it out" (Romans 7:18).

I'm struck by how much the Bible's wisdom about human dynamics continues to be backed up by modern neuroscience. Check out this description of what happens at the brain level when we're stressed:

> The amygdala activates stress pathways, which in turn impair prefrontal cortex regulation and strengthen amygdala function. This generates a vicious cycle in which high levels of stress keep the amygdala in the driver's seat. Our brain's response patterns switch from slow, thoughtful prefrontal cortex control to the reflexive and rapid emotional responses of the amygdala and related limbic structures. This explains why we become impulsive, irrational, and generally worse decision makers when we are stressed.[4]

To summarize, the more activated you are by stress and the less you're able to manage it, the more likely you are to make poor decisions. Chronic stress causes you to be reactionary (impulsive) instead of responsive (intentional). This very human instinct is designed for your survival, but over time, it can lead to poor decisions with unpleasant consequences. I believe this is the kind of dynamic Paul is describing when he says, "For I do not understand my own actions. For I do not do what I want, but I do the very thing I hate" (Romans 7:15).

Just to be clear, this isn't to say that being triggered is a sin. You are not a horrible person if you are emotionally activated by your environment. The fact that you get triggered is part of being human. However, sometimes your triggers can lead you to do things that you regret. On a micro level, you might overreact or explode on someone you love, using words you wish you could take back. On a macro level, you might engage in self-destructive behavior that leads to harming yourself or damaging relationships in ways you can't take back. I know how difficult it can be to determine if we made decisions based on a physiological disorder, trauma, or core beliefs. It's easy to beat yourself up for getting triggered and letting it show up in ways you wish you hadn't. I have been there—repeatedly—which is why I feel like Paul is speaking to me in Romans 7:15. But here's the thing I want you to remember: God can use your unwanted triggers to draw your attention to your need for emotional regulation—before that happens!

When we learn emotional regulation strategies, we can better access our prefrontal cortex to become more aware of our triggers, especially when they pop up in surprising ways. Here's an example of that: Years ago, after a gathering with my extended family, I found out through family gossip that another family member was holding resentment against me for an argument we had that weekend. Here's the thing: I had zero recollection of this argument. I tried everything I could to recall what had happened, and nothing came up. But hearing about the issue secondhand triggered me.

One of my biggest fears is getting in trouble or making someone mad at me. It's stress-inducing to my brain, so it's hard to tell my brain to work logically and get over it when I think someone doesn't like me. However, once I realized what was happening, I knew I had a choice—I could react (with brooding, passive-aggressive behavior or anger), or I could co-regulate. I chose to co-regulate by sharing my concerns with my husband, who was as dumbfounded about the situation as I was. He offered me comfort and empathy and helped me to see what bothered me wasn't the mystery argument itself, but how I thought I was perceived by the other person as a result. He gave me a second set of eyes, a helpful perspective, and his counsel allowed me to respond by letting it go, since the other party hadn't confronted me directly. Understanding triggers and learning to address them is an ongoing project for me, and I know I'm not alone.

What are your triggers? Perhaps you find yourself continuously worried about what people are saying or thinking about you. Or maybe you lie in bed at night, longing for sleep, but instead your brain is bouncing around, replaying difficult conversations; and all you can think about is how you should've said that one thing differently, or not said it at all. Perhaps you find yourself blowing up at your spouse or kids when the true cause of your anger is something else entirely. Or maybe you find yourself breaking down and crying after the tiniest amount of constructive criticism.

When you are constantly picking up on triggers, it can feel overwhelming. You may feel tightly wound, which causes you to mistrust your reactions under stress. But as someone who's been there, may I offer you some hope? Healthy emotional regulation is a skill you *can* master. And doing so begins with strengthening your emotional regulation muscles.

Strengthen Your Emotional Regulation

Strengthening your emotional regulation muscles is like a workout for your brain. It involves a few steps, including a warm-up, the workout itself, and the cooldown.

The warm-up. Become a student of your body and its symptoms. Use what you've learned and experienced about making mind-body connections to identify the signs that you're being triggered. For example, do you feel it in your body? If so, where? Do you experience being triggered as a rush of emotions? Or does it show up as one overwhelming emotion? When I'm triggered by an interruption or emotional discomfort, my whole body feels flooded with heat, and I start to sweat. The physical sensations clue me in that my brain has been alerted to danger in some way.

The workout. Now it's time to evaluate what your most common triggers are. A good way to do this is to recall the last time you got upset about something or with someone. Maybe, like in my example with the invisible family conflict, you're simply triggered by someone's misrepresentation of you. Or perhaps you got into an argument with your spouse about his failure to do something you asked him to do, and you were triggered because you felt disrespected. Or maybe one of your children threw a fit in public, and you were triggered because you worried others would judge you for your parenting failure. Whatever the situation was, reflect on and identify the reason for the trigger.

The cooldown. Create two lists. On one, write out all the things you might do that could help you to calm down when you're activated. Focus on the simple things you can do in the moment when you don't have time to completely pivot in your day. This could be butterfly taps, deep breathing, breath prayers, jumping jacks, walking away to regroup, or drinking a big glass of water.

On the other list, write down the preventative things you can do to strengthen your emotional regulation. What can you do throughout the week that helps you feel more regulated? I love asking my clients this question because the responses vary so much. Common answers include reading, walking, going to an exercise class, and being in nature. My client Laura loves yoga, cooking with music on, and spending time cuddling with her husband after the kids go to bed. Stephanie needs daily prayer and meditation to stay grounded. Another client loves to cross-stitch because it slows her breathing and allows her to focus on just the task at hand. Still another client loves to take baths and work in her garden. My friend Hannah recently told me she finds it stress-relieving to put together monster puzzles (just thinking about a puzzle builds up more stress for me). The point is, preventative regulation is individual, and the more you know what works for you, the more you can support your own regulation as needed.

Once you have your prevention list, take your self-check-in one step further. Estimate how much time you need to do the activities on your list each week. Write yourself a prescription for emotional regulation activities. My client Laura noticed there is a marked difference in her mental state when she is not going to yoga at least twice a week, so that is part of her prescription. Stephanie realized if she doesn't get her morning breath prayers in before she goes to work, she feels edgy. Even though her workdays are demanding, she sets a timer for three minutes every morning to pause and breathe through a Scripture passage.

Having a list of preventative regulation activities can also help you identify when you are feeling more reactionary than usual. When you become aware of your need for emotional regulation as well as your triggers, you can use your emotional regulation tools to recharge your batteries.

If you are struggling through a period of what feels like chronic triggering, I want you to know that you're not alone. These tools I share with you are not to bypass your pain. They're not cute ideas I came up with to fill a book. They have been anchors for me during the darkest storms in my life. My prayer is that you're able to use these tools to safely process your emotions and move forward. I offer them in hope that you will feel loved and supported just where you are, as you are—triggers and all.

MAKING THE MIND-BODY CONNECTION

If you struggle to identify your underlying emotions when triggered, this breathing-shift exercise, which I borrowed from my therapist husband, can help walk you through the process of identifying what triggers you so you can respond with healthy regulation. The purpose of the exercise is to use your body to regulate your emotions when you feel triggered.

- *Identify a memory that brings positive emotions (happiness, joy, peace, or safety).* Once you bring that memory to mind, notice how your body feels. It may feel like warmth is flowing through you, or you might feel more relaxed and less tense. Your chest may expand, giving you a lighter feeling, or your head might feel clearer. As you continue to focus on that memory, notice your breath: How fast is it? How deep is it? Then notice where your breath originates. Usually, a positive memory will cause your breath to come from your belly. Place your hand where your breath is coming from and keep it there.

- *Identify a memory that brings negative emotions (fear, anxiety, or sadness).* It might be a memory of a conflict, a frustration, or any other context in which you felt triggered. Don't choose anything too extreme, but find a memory with enough distress that you can pay attention to your body's response. Notice how your body changes as you bring up this memory. What sensations do you experience? You might notice your breathing shifts to a faster pace and becomes shallower; and it may move more to your chest. Your chest might feel tighter and more constricted, or your jaw may clench. If you notice your breathing shift to your chest, move your hand there in response.

- **Shift your breathing.** Keep your focus on the distressing memory, but shift your breathing to a slower, more regulated state. If you moved your hand to your chest, move it back to your belly and focus on breathing slowly and deeply from there instead of your chest. As you do, notice how your body changes your response to the memory. Notice how your sensations shift. You may feel calmer than before, and your body may feel less tense.

This exercise is an example of how you can use the body—through something as simple as a breathing shift—to bring calm to the mind.

14

MOVEMENT AS MEDICINE

Movement is incredible medicine for reestablishing the mind-body connection and creating stress resilience. However, when I ask clients about their relationship with exercise, I get varied responses. Some people love it and swear by it, but for others, finding a routine is intimidating. Even the word *exercise* can initiate shudders and bring up bad memories from PE class. For others, exercise creates a *dis*connect between mind and body; they do it because they "have to" instead of because they "want to." In my work with clients who struggle to integrate exercise in their health journeys, I've found that people generally fall into four different "types": *exercise hesitant, exercise dependent, exercise reluctant,* and *exercise punishing*. As you read the following examples, take mental notes on which type you relate to most.

Hailey knows she should exercise, and she knows she would feel better if she did, but she just can't seem to find something she likes enough to stick with it. She doesn't necessarily have a bad experience with exercise or even a bad relationship with it, but every time she attempts a consistent exercise routine, she quickly loses interest. In fact, at the start of the year she downloaded an exercise app and used it consistently, feeling great. Then one morning in February she found herself waffling between getting up or hitting snooze, so she hit snooze and slept longer. The next day, because of what happened the day before, she waffled again and once again chose to hit snooze. And just like that, she got out of the habit. She lacks intrinsic motivation, but if someone else encourages her or asks to join in, she will exercise—if she can fit it into her schedule. Hailey is *exercise hesitant*.

Deandra lives for exercise. She loves it, relies on it, and thrives when she's incorporating movement into her life. She loves how exercise supports her physically, whether to maintain weight, muscle, or health in general. She also benefits from the routine and consistency. In fact, it's the only time she has to herself the entire day. Unfortunately, she also shames herself for missing a workout. When she feels that she ruined her progress, she sees herself differently in the mirror, and then she makes plans to up the ante for the next workout. As a result, sometimes she experiences a robot-like attachment to exercise and finds herself completely ignoring discomfort that arises when she pushes herself too hard. When that happens, she chooses not to listen to her body but lives for the schedule—or the inner drill sergeant who criticizes her when she misses a workout. Deandra is *exercise dependent*.

Rita simply doesn't want to exercise. Deep down she knows she would benefit from it, and she likes the idea of exercise, but she's never felt comfortable enough in her skin to try different forms of movement. Exercise feels like an added task on top of so many other tasks that need to be done throughout the day. Working and raising young children, she has so many obligations, and the urgency of those tasks overpowers any desire to get out and intentionally move her body. She also feels silly to admit this, but she knows that committing to exercise will require finding the right sports bra or shoes, and even that task feels like an added hassle at this stage of life. She can't seem to justify fitting exercise into her life, though she knows it's a good thing. Rita is *exercise reluctant*.

Piper uses exercise to punish herself for food choices she made (or didn't make), and because she doesn't like the shape of her body or a particular body part. She likes to "burn to earn." She knows exercise is the right and healthy thing to do, so she takes it to the extreme and performs her movements with religiosity. At times, she pairs her exercise with rigid or restrictive dieting. She looks down on others who don't exercise as much as she does because they remind her of her own fear of not living up to the person she wants to be. When she exercises, she feels a deep but temporary sense of accomplishment, which means she's always oscillating between exercise accomplishment and exercise punishment—a vicious cycle. She's her own worst enemy, even though she believes that by exercising she is doing the best thing for herself and her body. Piper is *exercise punishing*.

Which of the examples do you resonate with most? I know I've experienced all four. My pattern was initially exercise reluctant (mostly because it's so dang hard to find a supportive sports bra); which led to being exercise hesitant and unable to find my routine; then exercise dependent once I did find my routine and wanted to maintain it; only to become exercise punishing to make up for my food choices.

It wasn't until I threw out my back multiple times that I was forced to wake up and view exercise differently. My lower back screamed at me several times before I decided to listen, but the final time was when I was halfway through my third pregnancy. I was determined to run throughout the pregnancy—I had even run a 15K at nine weeks pregnant (I don't know if that's punishment or foolishness). But my back said, *Nope!* That was the point at which I discovered yoga, and an entirely new perspective on exercise opened up for me.

I initially resisted the stillness and slow pace of yoga. I wanted to feel the accomplishment of a skyrocketing heart rate and lots of sweat. I wanted to feel like I was truly drowning out the noise of my thoughts and "burning" something off, as culture taught me was the best approach. The stillness and slow movement of yoga left me feeling uncomfortable and flat-out unsteady at first. However, it also forced me to be present for my body and my thoughts, despite how I felt about either of them. I had to breathe intentionally, instead of huffing and puffing to survive. I slowly began to view my body as a partner, not an enemy.

Eventually, I experienced a different level of relaxation than I did after heavy-duty cardio. I also experienced greater self-compassion and awareness. I adjusted my expectations of exercise based on what I truly needed, not what I thought I needed. By the time my back felt strong enough for me to reengage with high-impact movement, walking had become a new comfort. I no longer had the itch for more speed to prove something to myself, and I could enjoy movement for movement's sake. I saw the benefits of exercise for reasons other than obligation or body perfection. I was even able to stop tracking miles. I ran when I felt like running, and I walked when I felt like walking.

I was thirty-eight years old when I started truly listening to my body's needs through movement. To do that, I had to gain a fresh perspective on why I moved so I could create a habit that wasn't based on punishment or body criticism. I needed to reframe everything I ever told myself about exercise for weight loss or to earn permission to eat. And I discovered something interesting in the process. Specifically, I found that the benefits keeping me engaged in movement practices throughout the week were primarily about three things: igniting my brain, listening to my body, and connecting with God.

Movement Is a Way to Ignite Your Brain

When we hear about exercise benefits from magazines, fitness influencers, and celebrity trainers, we're hearing only about neck-down benefits, such as fitting into our clothes better. But the neck-up benefits—the mental health support—are the ones that make the most impact. When the brain is functioning better, everything is functioning better!

The first time I really considered movement's mental health benefits was when the character Elle Woods gave a mini-speech in *Legally Blonde* about endorphins from exercise making you feel good. (It's still one of my favorite movies.) Since then, I've learned that there are dozens of amazing processes that happen in the brain when we exercise. I've narrowed them down to my favorite three: brain-derived neurotrophic factor (BDNF), atrial natriuretic peptide (ANP), and neurotransmitter signaling. As usual, there won't be a quiz on the big words, but hold tight—you're going to be amazed at what movement does for the brain.

BDNF Is Your Brain's Miracle-Gro

Did you know that you aren't 100 percent stuck with the brain you have? Thanks to modern discoveries of neurogenesis (how the brain forms new neurons) and neuroplasticity (how the brain adapts to form new connections and pathways), we know the brain can change.

One change occurs with the exercise-induced release of brain-derived neurotrophic factor (BDNF). BDNF acts like Miracle-Gro for your brain's synapses, improving signaling. Here's what that means: Neurons are nerve cells in the brain. Picture a neuron as a tree with branches. Every branch is called a dendrite, and the leaves that form on the dendrites are synapses that strengthen connections between other neurons. BDNF strengthens those synaptic connections and encourages the neurons to communicate better by growing new branches (dendrites). As psychiatrist and researcher Dr. John Ratey writes, "BDNF gives the synapses the tools they need to take in information, process it, associate it, remember it, and put it in context."[1]

One of the reasons researchers believe exercise is such a potent antidepressant is because strengthening BDNF can improve mood. While elevated levels of the stress hormone cortisol decrease BDNF and lead to negative mood symptoms, exercise increases it. BDNF prevents cognitive decline by keeping our minds sharper over time. It's like a miracle serum for brain growth!

ANP Calms Your Response to Stress

I recently polled my Facebook friends and asked them, "If you exercise for reasons other than weight maintenance or body image, what are the benefits?" Multiple people commented that they felt calmer and more patient when they exercised. And guess what—there's a reason for that! It has to do with atrial natriuretic peptide (ANP).

ANP is produced by the heart muscle when it starts beating harder in response to movement. It travels through the blood and crosses into the blood-brain barrier, where it modulates the body's response to stress. It calms the HPA axis (which, if you recall, is the stress response system that alerts your body to fight, flight, freeze, or fawn). This results in an antianxiety effect.

Here's another really amazing fact, especially if you struggle with panic attacks: Panic attacks are known to stimulate the release of corticotropin-releasing factor (CRF), which tells the adrenal glands to release loads of cortisol into the bloodstream at once, leaving you with feelings of sudden panic. ANP puts the brakes on this release of CRF, resulting in a decrease in anxiety and panic. This is why a regular exercise routine can help you to feel more mentally regulated, calm, and patient.

Neurotransmitters Keep You Regulated

Neurotransmitters are chemical messengers, released from neurons, that move across synapses ("leaves" on the dendrite "tree branch") to bind to other neurons. Exercise causes the release of neurotransmitters, two of the most well-known being serotonin and dopamine. Serotonin is thought to be the "happy neurotransmitter" due to its antidepressant effects, but it also has anti-inflammatory effects and plays a large role in sleep and digestive regulation. Dopamine is the neurotransmitter that helps us with focus, learning, and motivation, and it's the reason we return to things we love—like a favorite exercise! In fact, getting a steady release of dopamine from exercise can help blunt cravings for substances that aren't health-promoting, such as hyperpalatable processed foods.[2] Both of these neurotransmitters are known to have mood-balancing effects.

Some less-known neurotransmitters that keep mood regulated and stable are called endocannabinoids. Endocannabinoids are released in the body from exercise, and they produce a drug-like effect (think "runner's high"). If you happened to connect the word "cannabis" to endocannabinoids, well done! Endocannabinoids are released when THC from marijuana binds to their receptors, but get this—exercise initiates the same release, to a lesser extent (don't worry, you're not going to fail a drug test). This leads to decreased perception of pain and a greater sense of calm.

There are other neurotransmitters that are released in response to exercise, such as GABA (a calming neurotransmitter), endorphins (feel-good chemicals), and acetylcholine (which regulates the gut-brain connection). The feel-good effects of exercise impact the brain's signaling of these messengers and flood the entire body with positive side effects.

Seeing all these benefits, it should come as no surprise to learn that a meta-analysis studying ninety-seven reviews and over one hundred thousand people determined that exercise is more than one and a half times more effective than talk therapy and medication in alleviating symptoms of depression, anxiety, and distress![3] That doesn't mean you should fire your therapist or quit your medication cold turkey and take up running instead. Please don't do that! However, it does scientifically demonstrate the brain-boosting benefits of movement.

When you find an exercise you enjoy and can make a habit, there are proven benefits for the brain. Choosing to move your body regularly in ways you enjoy also brings about another positive side effect: It helps you learn to listen to your body and attune to its needs.

Movement Is a Way to Listen to Your Body

The concept of using movement to tune in to the body's needs may seem strange, but it is so necessary in the healing journey. That's because movement is a powerful way to connect with your body by focusing on—yep, you've heard this before—partnership over punishment. In other words, it's *not* a formula for mind over matter. In fact, when you consistently put mind over matter at the expense of your body's needs, you're telling your body it doesn't matter. When you move your body in a way that feels good, you're giving it permission to communicate with you, which might not always have been the case, especially if you've struggled with chronic disease or mental illness, as my client Macy did.

Macy came to me for help managing her symptoms of bipolar disorder. In the fall months, she struggled with feelings of hypomania (elevated mood, increased goal-directed activity, lack of sleep, and rapid speech), and in the winter months with depression. Macy researched a lot about her illness, and she believed in the power of nutrition and movement for symptom management along with her prescribed medication. When it came to exercise, she found that in the fall, a regular routine helped her use up some of her excess energy and kept her balanced. However, as her mood dropped in the winter, so did her motivation to exercise. She felt like her body was working against her, and that made her angry with it, which perpetuated her low mood.

The more we talked, I noticed that Macy's bursts of exercise in the fall were reactionary to her symptoms, seen as a quick fix. She relied on exercise when she felt like it, and when she didn't feel like it anymore, she quit. I helped her to see that exercise could work as a preventative tool as well as for in-the-moment support. Over time, she was able to develop a routine that she stuck to for the long-term benefits, not just the short-term results; but she had to change it up according to her body's needs. While her fall workouts were fueled with high-intensity training, her needs in winter shifted to long walks and restorative yoga, where she had to slow down and breathe intentionally through her movements. Consistently moving during the winter months in a different way helped to get her out of the "freeze state" in which she found herself. It allowed her to listen to the fluctuation of her body and adjust accordingly.

Rachel came to me for support with her fluctuating hormones. At forty-one, she was experiencing early symptoms of perimenopause, which left her with drastic mood changes before her period, low energy and brain fog, sudden belly weight, and body aches she'd never experienced before. She already had an exercise routine, along with a healthy relationship with exercise, but her body's changing symptoms freaked her out. She started working out at a greater intensity and for a longer duration, yet her symptoms remained. I explained that the female body has four distinct phases during a month, and certain life stages such as perimenopause make those phases more sensitive to any stress—even good stress such as exercise. When she adjusted her workouts according to her cycle and her body's needs, her symptoms leveled out.

Exercise is a way to adapt to your body's needs by tuning in and listening; it's not just a box to check off on the to-do list. When you engage with your body by listening to it, it's a gift for the mind-body connection. It creates a partnership and strengthens signaling so you are more aware of how to adjust your lifestyle to become stronger and more resilient to stress.

However, too much of a good thing, including exercise, can still be too much. Remember from chapter 2, exercise is considered a *hormetic stressor*. That means it is designed to put your body through stress for a short period and then allow time for recovery. The assumption is that you *can* recover from it. That's not always the case.

Imagine this scenario: You jump right out of bed for your pre-workout caffeine (stress), to your intense workout (stress), to racing to get ready for the day (stress). By the time you get to work or start your daily routine of household duties and caretaking (or both), you've already depleted some of your stress reserves and have little to no margin for recovery—unless you consider your recovery time to be a streaming app and a glass of wine at the end of the day (screen stress and liquid stress). Then if you're lucky, you get a halfway decent night's sleep so you can perpetuate the cycle all over again.

Do you see how exercise might be adding one more block to the tower of stress in your life? If you're not consistently sleeping well, if you feel fatigue throughout the day, if your exercise habit makes you more irritable than anything else, or if you experience changes in your menstrual cycle or digestive regularity, it might be time to consider adjusting your movement to your current season of life. Instead of high intensity, switch to low impact, such as walking or body weight training (Pilates, barre, or yoga).

The way you move your body and the information you give it during a workout can impact the benefits you get from it. If you're exercising merely as a performance or obligation, and you're gritting your teeth to make it through, your body picks up on that. That's no longer a positive hormetic stressor; it's acute disruptive stress! If you're moving in ways you enjoy, while also feeling a healthy challenge to keep going, that builds resilience. That's a good thing.

For me, this means staying away from group sports. I have many friends who play tennis, and I really wanted to enjoy tennis; but (surprise, surprise) I hate letting other people down by my mistakes. I prefer individual workouts. I'm intrinsically motivated, so I'll run if I feel like it, challenging myself to a few minutes of sprinting throughout. Or I'll lift weights and challenge myself to a few extra reps. In yoga, even though I'm with others, my challenge is to be present with my body and focus on gratitude for how it supports me. These noncompetitive individual workouts, while challenging in the moment, allow me to listen to my body's needs and partner with it while also giving me a feeling of accomplishment when I finish.

You might be the opposite of me. Maybe movement is a way you can socialize and receive nourishment from a source of primary nourishment, your relationships with others. However you decide to move your body, using movement to tune in to your body's needs is a powerful tool for your healing journey and a way to empower yourself to be your own health advocate. And, if you're anything like me, you may find that your favorite aspect of movement comes from the way it enables you to connect with God.

Cycle Sync Your Workouts

If you have an active menstrual cycle, your body experiences constant change throughout the month (even your brain changes volume depending on what phase of your cycle you're in). Cycle syncing your workouts can be a great way to connect with your body and listen to its needs. Here's what that looks like according to each phase:

Follicular phase (roughly seven to ten days). This phase occurs right after menstrual bleeding ends. All sex hormones (progesterone, estrogen, testosterone, follicle-stimulating hormone, and luteinizing hormone) are at low levels and slowly start to increase. With the hormone increase comes an energy increase for most. Use this energy to enjoy movements that are fast-paced and fun for you, such as dance, cardio, high-intensity interval training (HIIT), or strength training.

Ovulatory phase (three to four days). The hormone rise continues, stimulating egg release. This is accompanied by a surge in testosterone, which increases desire and motivation. Many women are more sociable during this phase. The heightened energy lends itself to higher intensity workouts, and it's a great time to try group fitness classes because the group dynamic will fuel your energy even more.

Luteal phase (ten to fourteen days). During the first part of this phase, energy remains high, but as hormones drop before menstruation, so will your energy and stress tolerance. Use this time to tune in to your body's needs and scale back your workouts to calmer activities such as walking, Pilates, yoga, and light strength training.

Menstrual phase (three to seven days). All sex hormones drop to their lowest concentration as your body sheds the lining of the uterus. It's completely okay to hit snooze or consider a nap after your workout if you need to. Toward the end of the phase, pay attention to increasing energy and use that to do what makes your body feel best.

For more support on cycle syncing, download the MyFlo app.

Movement Is a Way to Connect with Your Creator

You've been given one vessel to live out your God-given purpose. I know your vessel may not have arrived in the package you wanted, and the symptoms it gives you don't seem necessary; but it *is* part of the three-in-one design (body-mind-spirit) that mirrors the three-in-one God (Father-Son-Spirit) who created you. As humans, we have a gift that no other created being has: being made in the image of God. As an image-bearer, you can use your physical body to both connect with God and to live out your purpose.

Your body is a conduit of God's love for the world. "The physical part of you is not some piece of property belonging to the spiritual part of you," wrote the apostle Paul. "God owns the whole works. So let people see God in and through your body" (1 Corinthians 6:19-20, MSG). The way you care for others is demonstrated through your physical body—for example, in how you rush to pick up a fallen child, reach out your arms to embrace a hurting friend, and dance for joy at a wedding reception.

Likewise, when you move your body in the way it was designed to move, and do so for fun, it activates a greater connection with your purpose. Did you know that myokines, proteins manufactured in muscles and released into the bloodstream during physical activity, were called "hope molecules" in early research studies? When you contract your muscles in movement, myokines are released past the blood-brain barrier to improve mood and learning, creating an effect known as "muscle-brain cross-talk."[4] These hope molecules help to increase mind-body communication. This increase in mental clarity can also increase communication with the needs of your soul—your communication with your heavenly Father.

While you may be accustomed to partnering with your mind or spirit to connect with God, the idea that you can also partner with your body to connect with God may initially seem hard to believe. I grew up in a faith-based home, so praying was something I did daily. Asking God for help with self-control, patience, and other challenging character qualities was common. Asking God to remind me to use my body to connect with him? Not so common.

However, some of the greatest aha moments in my spiritual journey have come during long walks or yoga class, when I chose to use that time to worship. When I lie in "corpse pose" at the end of a yoga class, my palms facing upward, I use that posture to offer my whole self to God. When I walk up the steep hill behind my house, I pump my legs and arms in gratitude for the adrenaline burst that keeps me going. When I finish a difficult round of weights, I am reminded that I can persist during difficulty and grow from it. During times in my life when I can't sit still or focus, listening to reminders of his faithfulness via worship music on a walk or in yoga helps me to connect with truth in a way I wouldn't be able to absorb as easily if I were sitting still.

Movement brings hope. It reminds us that our bodies are vessels, dwelling places for the Holy Spirit, whom Jesus described as our "Advocate" or "Helper" (see John 14:26, ESV, NIV). When our movement produces endorphins, dopamine, and even the hope molecules called myokines, we not only affirm the mind-body connection but also the soul-body connection that enables us to be present to God and live with hopeful purpose on earth.

MAKING THE MIND-BODY CONNECTION

There are three types of movement I often recommend to my clients, both for the health benefits and for enjoyment: Zone 2 cardio, strength training, and mobility/flexibility training. Here are some easy ways to practice all three.

- *Zone 2 cardio.* This is any type of exercise that gets your heart rate up to 60–70 percent of its maximum rate, which means you should be able to carry on a conversation with another person while moving at a low intensity. You can calculate your maximum heart rate by subtracting your age from 220, then calculating 60 percent of that number. For example, if you're forty, your zone 2 heart rate is

60 percent of 180, which is 108 beats per minute. Ideally, you want to get 150 minutes of zone 2 cardio in one week, which works out to just over twenty minutes a day, seven days a week (or thirty minutes a day, five days a week). Walking on a slight incline is one way to achieve your zone 2 cardio heart rate. Recent studies show that adding just 500 to 1,000 steps per day reduces your mortality risk, so I consider it the most underrated free tool for health.[5]

- *Strength training.* Strength training, which is also called weight or resistance training, uses weights and resistance devices to increase muscle strength and develop strong bones. Building muscle is protective for both the brain and body. Strength training two to three times a week is optimal, but there's no rule. If you're just starting out, there are many free tutorials online for beginners, and all you need is a set of hand weights. To protect against injury, it's important to have the right form. If you're just beginning your strength training journey, it might be helpful to watch videos or hire a fitness trainer to make sure you're using the right form.

- *Mobility/flexibility training.* One of my favorite forms of mobility training is restorative yoga, which focuses on stretching, deep breathing, and calming the nervous system. My friend Luci is a yoga therapist, and her motto is, "Practice with the body you have today." During high stress weeks or seasons, or depending on where you are in your menstrual cycle, you may need to simply stretch and breathe, and restorative yoga is a helpful tool to remind the body to enter a parasympathetic (rest-and-digest) state. There are many videos available online to help you get started.

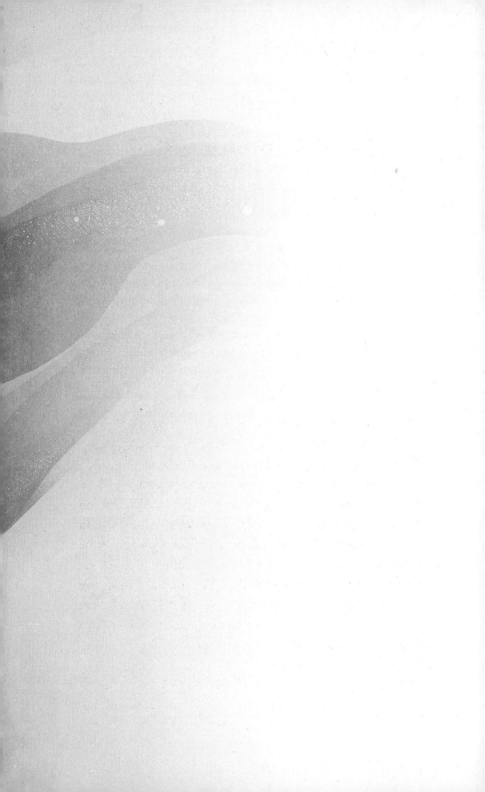

15

HEALING THROUGH REST

"Tell me about your sleep. What's it like?" I asked my new client Alexis, a mom of two school-age children. She'd sought out my help regarding her recent autoimmune disease diagnosis.

"I try to have a consistent sleep schedule," she sighed. "I do okay for the most part. But there's always something I have to do last minute before bed, like making sure my kids' uniforms are in the laundry room and not in a pile on their floor. Or we get home late from soccer practice, and by the time I sit down to eat dinner, it's 8:30. I need time after that to chill. There's always something else I'm forgetting or needing to catch up on. It's a busy season right now because the kids are involved in so many things. When I do sleep, I guess it's fine. But I don't know if I really feel rested. It's like my brain is always awake."

"What do you do for rest or self-care?" I asked.

"I mean, I get a pedicure like once a month or so," she said.

"Do you make time for stillness or meditation, that kind of thing?" I asked.

She laughed. "If I get too still, I'll probably fall asleep. I need to stay in motion, or it'll all fall apart."

I nodded, wondering how to gently phrase my next comment. "Well, it makes me wonder if part of the reason your body is screaming at you for attention is because it's not getting the rest it needs. The things that work for us to manage stress work well . . . until they don't. Sometimes we need new solutions."

"I get that," she sighed. "And I feel that in my whole body, but it's so hard to stay afloat right now. There's always something else I need to deal with."

Do you ever feel like Alexis does? *There's always something else.* Right when you think you can take two steps forward in one life season, you're taking one step back because another season brings unexpected changes. Then when you think you're in the clear, managing this season well, there's another mini-emergency. Or an alert. Or something urgent that must be attended to. It leaves you with a "wired but tired" feeling that many in our culture have come to view as normal. However, it's exhausting, and if you resonate, you're not alone.

According to the World Health Organization, which publishes the *International Classification of Diseases,* burnout is classified as an "occupational phenomenon" and defined as "a syndrome conceptualized as resulting from chronic workplace stress that has not been successfully managed."[1] People all over the world are struggling with lack of motivation and energy in the workplace, and I'd argue that burnout extends far beyond the work environment, especially in recent years. I've sat with many women and men who are experiencing parenting burnout, ministry or volunteer burnout, and even marriage burnout as they can't seem to keep up with the daily pressures they put upon themselves.

When you're doing everything for everyone else and have very little time to manage your own rest and relaxation practices, burnout will inevitably follow. And when you're burned out, rest becomes reactionary (a state your nervous system forces you into) rather than responsive (a state you choose when you know you're starting to feel slightly overwhelmed). That's when finding restful sleep starts to feel like entering an obstacle course every night when you get into bed. As I've said, your body won't heal in a sympathetic-dominant state of rushing. You need rest to heal. To support your body's unique need for rest, you first must establish an intentional self-care practice. And self-care probably looks a little different than what you might expect.

Self-Care Acknowledges Your Need for Rest

What's the first image that pops into your mind when you hear the term *self-care*? If it's something like getting your nails done or having a spa day, you're not alone. That's what Alexis thought too! While there's nothing wrong with either of those, they aren't what I mean when I talk about the importance of self-care. Self-care is the practice of acknowledging your need for rest and doing whatever you can to make time for it. It is choosing purposeful activities to meet the need for rest and balance in your body, mind, and spirit.

Self-care springs from self-awareness. For me, that means knowing my limits and putting protections in place so I don't ever exceed full capacity. When I exceed my capacity, I crash. So it's important for me to make time in my week for stillness and to avoid overscheduling my weekends. That ensures that I have "breathing room" to replenish myself no matter how busy my week gets or how my responsibilities shift.

Although we tend to think of self-care as a modern indulgence, it's actually an ancient practice—and a biblical one. The biblical foundation is in the principles of stewardship and discernment. Your body is God's gift to you, and taking time to care for your physical needs is being a good steward of what you've been given. Self-care also involves partnering with the Holy Spirit in discernment to know your body's limits. Discernment is what helps you know it's time to take a break. And can you guess who in the Bible modeled this well? Jesus himself.

There are multiple examples in Scripture of Jesus making time for intentional rest. He took breaks to recharge and "would withdraw to desolate places and pray" (Luke 5:16). After the disciples returned from a busy ministry mission, Jesus instructed them to find a quiet place and rest awhile (Mark 6:30-31). When Jesus visited with Mary and Martha, Martha was caught up in rushing and doing, distracted by her service; but Mary sat at Jesus' feet and listened to him. When Martha complained to Jesus about her sister, Jesus responded, "Martha, Martha, . . . you are worried and upset about many things, but few things are needed—or indeed only one. Mary has chosen what is better, and it will not be taken away from her" (Luke 10:41-42, NIV). In both his life and his teaching, Jesus affirmed the importance of intentional rest and quiet.

The danger in not making time for restorative self-care is that burnout and exhaustion can often lead to self-medication. Self-medication is the opposite of self-care. It happens when you decide *not* to listen to the still small voice reminding you to slow down and instead listen to the voice of productivity telling you to keep going because people are depending on you. Then you make a crash landing on the couch, where you spend the remaining hours of the day mindlessly scrolling through social media or binge-watching shows on a streaming service. While self-care allows you to partner with your body for rest, self-medication requires you to separate yourself from your body and check out. If you're

Intentional Self-Care Practices to Bring Rest to the Body

Here are some self-care ideas you can use to pause from the hurried pace of life and routinely give your body opportunities to rest and refresh:

- Spend fifteen minutes doing something that brings you peace and that doesn't involve a screen. It might be reading a book or magazine, journaling, crafting, taking a relaxing bath, gardening, or moving in nature.
- Take a twenty-four-hour screen break. Turn off all phone notifications. Spend time with people and activities you love.
- Each night before bed, practice a "brain dump" and write about your highs and lows for the day. Check in with your feelings. If you find it helpful, use the Examen prayer from chapter 8 (page 125).
- Spend time with people you care about at least once a week, engaging in conversation and fun. Laughter is an incredible de-stressing tool. Intentional community prevents feelings of isolation.
- Take a nap. Seriously. Lie down for twenty minutes. If you fall asleep, great. If not, you still gave your body an intentional break it will be grateful for.
- Make your favorite meal. Before sitting down to enjoy it, take a few deep breaths in through your nose and let them out through your mouth. Close your eyes and say a prayer of gratitude to God, who is your primary source of nourishment.
- If you're a parent, be intentional about your children's activities. Instead of signing them up for every activity (which ends up hijacking the family calendar), give them the option to choose one activity a season. Set boundaries with the activity schedule so you can model restful self-care to them.
- Choose one of the mind-body activities listed at the end of the previous chapters to incorporate into your day for seven consecutive days.

wondering how to determine whether an activity is self-care or self-medication, the best way I know how to distinguish them is this: *Self-care is proactive, and self-medication is reactive.* In other words, self-care helps you attune to your need for rest, and self-medication cuts you off from your deepest needs.

While *self-medication* often makes people think of substance abuse, the kind of reactionary self-medication I'm talking about can also happen from neutral or even seemingly positive behaviors. It might be saying yes to every volunteer opportunity—even though you're exhausted—because you have a desire to feel needed and appreciated. It might look like shopping as a distraction, or bingeing Netflix until hours past your bedtime. It could be eating half a bag of chips before you realize what you're even doing or how you got to the pantry. It may take the form of spending all your time going and doing so you don't have to sit in silence or solitude, because reflecting on your own needs feels uncomfortable and anxiety-producing. Self-medication comes from a natural desire to fill up when you're depleted, except you're filling up on the things that leave you empty.

If you're a chronic overscheduler and to-do list maker, the idea that you need to prioritize rest and self-care may be hard to hear, but think of it this way: Establishing a regular practice of rest makes you more efficient with the other tasks you need to do. Not only that, but doing all you need to do from a place of rest rather than exhaustion creates more intention and purpose than running on autopilot, which is a precursor to burnout. It's a crucial component of healing.

Relaxation and Rest Create Space to Pause

The practice of intentional relaxation and rest goes back all the way to the story of Creation itself, when God "rested from all his work"

(Genesis 2:2, NIV). The word *Sabbath* literally means "to stop." When we rest on the Sabbath, we stop going, stop doing, stop achieving, stop seeking, and stop running on autopilot. If the God of the universe thought it was important to devote a day to rest after creating the whole world in six days, we, too, can prioritize rest. God set an example for us when he chose to rest because rest is an essential part of what makes creation and our lives good. Going against this creation pattern by refusing to take a day of rest puts our lives out of balance—mentally, physically, and spiritually. An intentional pause makes space for awareness and growth.

When we choose to make rest first rather than last, we acknowledge that we have enough and we are enough, just as we are, without the hustle. That may be a difficult truth to accept for some of us achievers in the room, am I right? Choosing to stop also means we can rest in the knowledge that our true source of rest and healing comes from our Creator. It is a way to "be still, and know" that he is God and he is in control, even when we are resting (Psalm 46:10).

Making time for relaxation practices is something I require for all my clients, often before we even focus on nutrition or movement practices. I encouraged my client, Alexis, who was struggling with autoimmune disease, to spend ten hours a day intentionally resting. That didn't mean ten hours of sleep; it meant getting into bed early to read and wind down or waking up early to journal and start with a slow morning instead of rushing to her high-intensity workout class.

I encourage you to make time for days of rest. Given everything you likely need to do and accomplish in a week, I know this may seem like an impossibility, but you must make time to slow down. Your pace of life matters to your brain and body, and when it's unrelenting, it can negatively impact your ability to rest. Perhaps start small by having an enjoyable meal around the table instead of fast food in the car on the way to your next event.

Perhaps allow the laundry to pile up for one more day so you can take the evening off from household chores. Review your calendar for the weeks ahead and begin planning now to do things differently for the sake of your physical, emotional, and spiritual health.

Setting up healthy boundaries that enable you to have responsive rest is not selfish. It's a way to connect to the needs of your body. Choosing to quiet your mind by stepping away from the constant activity of daily life is not disengaging or dissociating. It's protecting your purpose. And get this: When you make space to rest regularly, your sleep patterns will improve as a result. Even though rest is not the same thing as sleep, making time for intentional moments of rest throughout your week, or taking an entire day off, reminds your brain there *is* an off switch. Rest and sleep feed off each other. When you rest well, your brain feels safer to activate healing sleep. When you sleep well, you have better impulse control and can make clearer decisions to rest. Supporting sleep habits is crucial for creating more habits of rest.

Sleep Support Starts During the Day

There are so many ways to support a good night's sleep, and the studies confirm—we need it! Over 30 percent of adults get less than the recommended seven hours of sleep each night.[2] According to the CDC, 14.5 percent of adults have trouble falling asleep, and 17.8 percent have trouble staying asleep.[3] If that seems like no big deal, consider that just one poor night of sleep can negatively impact learning, concentration, energy, mood, immune system strength, and eating habits the following day. While that information may not shock you, it might surprise you to learn that what you do during the day impacts how you sleep at night. Here are three things you can do during your day to support a good night's rest. While these guidelines may seem basic, I've learned that sometimes it's the most basic things that are hardest to implement. And yet, they're also the ones that have the potential to make the greatest impact when practiced consistently over time.

Increase exposure to natural light. To prime your circadian clock (which regulates the sleep-wake cycle), try getting morning sunlight in your eyes within thirty minutes of waking. This can support the production of melatonin twelve to fourteen hours later. If getting morning sunlight isn't possible for you, that's okay. Neuroscientist Andrew Huberman suggests that "afternoon sunlight serves as a second 'anchor point' for your brain and body to know the time/season, in order to maintain the consistency of your circadian clock."[4]

Natural sunlight makes a difference in sleep. When you consider that for most of human history we lived without electricity, artificial indoor light is a relatively new phenomenon for the human body. As a result, you and I live in flip-flopped times when we're exposed to less bright light during the day and more bright light at night. It's very confusing to our natural circadian balance, and it can negatively impact sleep patterns. This was a game changer for my client, Lisa, who had "tried everything" for her sleep. We changed up her supplements and evening routine, which helped some. But the most noticeable shift happened when she began exposing her eyes to morning sun, consistently (not just one time). Within weeks, she was sleeping more deeply and waking up feeling rested.

Engage in regular physical activity. Not getting enough physical activity during the day hinders optimal sleep at night. Want to prime your circadian clock and get movement in at the same time? Get your morning sun exposure on a morning walk. The stress hormone cortisol peaks in the morning, then tapers down throughout the day, giving rise to melatonin (a hormone that is produced when it gets dark and that supports sleep). Exercising early in the day to match the natural production of cortisol helps to engage the body and brain. It's a way to reassure the body that as the day progresses, so will activity. For that reason, it's best to avoid intense exercise within three to five hours of bedtime. It might hinder melatonin production.

Limit caffeine consumption. The amount of caffeine you consume during the day can impact how rested you feel at night. The caffeine conversation is always a fun one to have with clients, because it truly is individual. Some people metabolize caffeine quickly and others more slowly. The average half-life of caffeine metabolism (the amount of time it takes for half the caffeine to be used up) ranges from about five to seven hours,[5] but it can vary depending on the person. That could mean that if you have coffee at 3:00 p.m. to get through your afternoon slump, you'll still have half the caffeine in your system by 10:00 p.m. when you're supposed to be winding down for bed. For optimal sleep support, I always encourage clients to cut off caffeine at noon, or at least by 2:00 p.m.

In addition to adjusting daytime habits, the environment you surround yourself with and the practices you put into place just hours before you shut your eyes can also impact the way you sleep.

Sleep Hygiene Helps You to Wind Down

The practice of *how* you wind down makes a big difference in the quality of sleep you receive and how rested you feel when you wake up. Sleep hygiene is a cutesy term that simply means the practices and habits you use to create an environment for restful sleep. The following healthy sleep habits can help you optimize your sleep.

Adjust the lighting. Dim the lights in your home when it gets dark outside by turning off overhead lights you aren't actively using and utilizing soft lamplight instead. Eliminate all exposure to lights from screens and electronic devices from 10:00 p.m. to 4:00 a.m. Wear blue-light blocker glasses while using screens after dark, especially if you have light-colored eyes (you may be more sensitive to light). The blue light from screens and even LED lightbulbs suppress melatonin production.

Create an environment of absolute darkness in your bedroom. Block the numbers on the bedside clock (if you still have one). Keep your electronics (phone, tablet, computer) in another room to avoid interruptions. Use blackout curtains. If that's not possible, use a sleep mask.

Create a sound barrier. Depending on where you live, it may be beneficial to minimize external noise while you sleep by using a white noise machine, or a ceiling or box fan. This will keep you in a cocoon of neutral sound. If you find white noise disruptive rather than relaxing, try to find other ways to limit any extra noise so you can keep your body in an undisturbed state while you sleep.

Improve air quality. Some people struggle with restful sleep due to allergies, which may be triggered by dust mites, pet dander, air filters that need to be changed, or seasonal changes; and histamine release in response to those allergens can peak while you sleep, as it follows the circadian rhythm.[6] There are many ways to improve air quality, such as changing air filters (if you have central heating and air) every three months, adding indoor plants, changing bedding weekly, utilizing an air purifier, or dusting and vacuuming regularly.

Mind the temperature. Keep the temperature fairly cool, around sixty-eight degrees for optimal sleep support. While that may seem too cold for you, some researchers say that sixty-five degrees is the preferred temperature, because "to successfully initiate sleep . . . your core temperature needs to decrease by 2 to 3 degrees Fahrenheit."[7]

Unwind with a warm bath. When you get out of the bath, the drop in body temperature can lead to a natural sleepiness. Use Epsom salts in your bath if you're having a particularly stressful day. Epsom salts contain magnesium, so it's a great way to get the calming effects of the mineral magnesium through your skin. Stick to pure Epsom salts that are fragrance-free. You can add a few drops of a calming essential oil if you'd like.

Solidify your routine. Maintain the same bedtime every night, within about an hour window. Set an alarm on your phone at night for when you want to start winding down. Keep the same waketime—even on weekends. Sleeping later on weekends can make it more difficult to get up when Monday rolls around. The body prefers a consistent rhythm.

Avoid stressful shows or movies before bed (this includes the news). Watching a stress-inducing program can activate the nervous system into a sympathetic state of fight, flight, freeze, or fawn—even if it's for entertainment. It's yet another reminder that your body responds the same way to both real and perceived stress.

Avoid food and alcohol within two to three hours of sleeping. Eating before bed can disrupt the detoxification processes your body goes through at night and may lead to indigestion. Alcohol might feel calming in the moment, due to the increase in the production of the calming neurotransmitter GABA. However, the body compensates for the GABA release with a surge of excitatory neurotransmitter glutamate in the middle of the night, which can lead to an increase in anxiety-driven insomnia.

Don't miss your sleep bus. You know that feeling. You're reclining on the couch after a long day, watching another episode of that nineties sitcom that brings you comfort, and your eyelids start to feel heavy. When that happens, your sleep bus is approaching. Get off the couch and start your bedtime routine. If you push through and continue watching the show, you may get a second wind, which is a surge of cortisol, and you don't need that.

Calm your mind. Let out the day's stress by practicing a few rounds of breath prayers (page 67), or try the 4-7-8 breathing activity (page 77) when you first lie down. Or, before your head hits the pillow, journal or "brain dump" on paper to let go of the day's events. Detox your mind of the day's stressors and let it all out, through words on a page or breath work.

Creating an environment for deep, restful sleep reminds your body that it can activate the parasympathetic state of the nervous system, which lets it know it is safe to heal. Likewise, practicing habits of intentional rest and slowing down to recharge reminds the body that it doesn't have to be in survival mode all the time.

As a reminder, choosing rest isn't lazy. It isn't tapping out or giving up. It's simply giving yourself permission to tend to the needs of your body. Healing won't happen in a state of hurry. Healing will happen when you provide the nourishment your mind and body crave—and when you create an environment to rest and receive it.

MAKING THE MIND-BODY CONNECTION

Non-sleep deep rest (NSDR), a phrase coined by Stanford neuroscience professor Dr. Andrew Huberman, is a gentle, guided body scan that keeps your brain in a calm state, while slowing down brain waves, similar to sleep.[8] Practicing a ten-minute session of NSDR can engage the brain in a restful state, lead it into more focus later, and ultimately promote deeper sleep at night.

Try this guided practice if you're struggling to get to sleep or if you wake up in the middle of the night.

- Lying flat on your back in your bed with your hands at your sides, slowly inhale through your nose and exhale through your mouth, feeling your body relax and melt into your bed. Practice breathing in and out effortlessly, releasing all tension.

- Starting with the right side of your body, contract and release the muscles in areas of your body. Start with your head and neck, and then move progressively downward to your shoulders, arms, hands, chest, abdomen, hip, thigh, knee, calves, feet, and toes. Then work your way back up, contracting and releasing, bringing awareness to each body part and actively relaxing it as you inhale and exhale.

- Repeat the same contracting and releasing process on the left side of your body.

The goal is to create awareness of your body, breathing through various parts to create a sense of relaxation throughout in preparation for sleep.

Labeled with Wholeness

I hope you see how identifying and examining your labels are necessary parts of the journey to wholeness. I hope you understand how assembling the puzzle pieces that make you who you are is a catalyst that brings deeper connections within yourself and to the world around you. And I hope you know that your label doesn't define you or leave you trapped in a life of compartmentalized limitations. I hope you feel equipped to live a life of connection—mind, body, and spirit.

My greatest desire for you is that by journeying through these pages with me, you've realized that you're not alone in your overwhelm, anxiety, depression, negativity, trauma, emotional outbursts, or seemingly dysregulated habits. Your body and brain aren't broken but are working together—for you—to keep you moving forward into your purpose. I hope you understand how your body provides alerts to draw you closer to the Lord and that you are motivated to seek his wisdom in how to care for it. God designed your body with interconnections that are ultimately meant to point you back to him. Your holistic interconnectedness is part of your miraculous design. By integrating nourishment for your whole self through learning to address stress, identifying root issues, adding variety to your diet, and exercising your body and brain, you can walk in the newness of abundant life.

As you take your next steps to live beyond your label, receive these words as my blessing for your journey:

> *May you see your body as whole*
> > *and feel nourished by your Creator's presence wherever you go.*
>
> *May peace be with your body—*
> > *your feet that have traveled rocky paths, searching for grounding and stability,*
> > *your hands that have reached out for connection,*
> > *your belly that has felt the stirring of every Big Feeling within it,*
> > *your heart that beats—and holds all your hurts and longings.*
>
> *May peace be with your mind—*
> > *your questions and your need to understand,*
> > *your broken places,*
> > *your stress signals that propel you to seek healing.*
>
> *May peace be with your spirit—*
> > *your endless search for safety,*
> > *your desire for the Almighty God to hear you,*
> > *your inmost being, which longs for shalom.*
>
> *May you nourish yourself well.*
> *May you be reminded to take a breath and pause.*
> *May you listen to the alerts your body gives you.*
> *May you be filled with gentleness and compassion for the person you were and are.*
> *May you know that there is more to your story than the struggles of your body and brain,*
> > *that you have been designed for wholeness.*
>
> *May the peace that passes understanding fill your body, mind, and spirit,*

LABELED WITH WHOLENESS

and may that peace sustain you with the knowledge that you are not your label.
You are not your past.
You are not your faulty core beliefs.
You are whole.

Acknowledgments

This book is the culmination of a forty-year dream that started when I was four and told my mom I would one day be a writer. Because of that, I have a lifetime of people to thank.

I am grateful to my family, beginning with Richard, the love of my life. You are still my triple threat, keeping me grounded in mind, body, and spirit. Thank you for reminding me I'm not too much for you—or for God. Thank you for listening to my dreams and shutting down my inner critic when she pops up to boss me around. And thanks for reading and offering your professional therapist opinion (even on your days off). Isabel, you are the first best thing that happened to me. I'm so proud of the woman you've become and how you're using your unique brain to fight for those who need someone to fight for them. Thank you for letting me share your miraculous birth story. Roman, you are a grounding presence, like your daddy, and your encouragement and excitement in this publishing process shows me glimpses of the incredible young man you'll become. Rhett, your imaginative brain and constant questions keep me on my toes, reminding me how fun it is to ask, *Why?* Your ability to dream out loud inspires us all.

My parents: Dad, I wanted to be you when I was little. You're the ultimate wordologist, but it's the way you engage people and

ACKNOWLEDGMENTS

make them feel seen that has impacted me most. Mom, you stayed beside me during the darkest times, even at the expense of your own mental well-being. I'll never fully understand what you sacrificed, but I'm so grateful you did. Thanks for never giving up.

Jordan and Jess: Your support and excitement fueled me on this journey. Jordan, thank you for never being afraid of feeling out loud. Jessica, thank you for the verses of encouragement, always sent when I needed them.

Mammoo: I did it! I wrote a real book. I can't wait to talk to you about this one day in heaven. Thank you for taking me to the library instead of sending me fishing with PopPop. We shared so many words together. I know there will be more to come.

My extended Kerry family: Thank you for your support and continuous love.

My agent, Bob Hostetler: Thank you for taking a chance on me! You've been so helpful in this process, especially when I'm (maybe, kind of a little bit) starting to freak out and overthink things.

My acquiring editor, Jillian Schlossberg: Thank you for supporting the vision for this work and the beautiful interconnectedness of functional medicine and the Bible.

My publisher, Jan Long Harris: It's still surreal to me that you invited me to be part of the Tyndale Refresh imprint. Thank you for the opportunity to share my passion.

My editor, Christine Anderson: You are my brain's translator, and your magic touch made the manuscript so much more structured and connected. (Also, thanks for giving me freedom to create sidebars—and parentheses, like this one—when I had one more thought to add.)

My copy editor and fact-checker, Elizabeth Czajkowski: Thank you for your eye for details and your suggestions that gave this book the ultimate glow-up.

The entire Tyndale team: You are the village who helped raise my book baby, and I'm so grateful!

My mentor Sandra Beck: Your coaching pushed me forward. You encouraged me to start my podcast and take a chance. Thank you for believing in me.

My friend Heather Creekmore: This book wouldn't exist if you hadn't told me to send in a proposal. Your wisdom and guidance changed the game!

The TogiNet podcast production team—Scott Frazier, Ben Horlander, and Roy Bryant: Thank you for getting my podcast out into the world and helping me troubleshoot the technology (and Apple issues).

Bismark, my assistant: Thank you for keeping my podcast calendar straightened out and reminding me to send the newsletter!

Beta readers of the first version—Luci Davis, Lauren Gossett, Mori Randal, Lori Harris, Janet Van Dam, Rachel Wilson, Jennie Sage, Ann Terese Brandt, Kayla Hefner, Dafne Vargas, Leslie Bateman, Lindsay Berryman, Annie Corrales, and Katie Butts: Thank you for offering your constructive feedback on the very early version of this book. Bobi Ann Allen, thank you for the detailed markups and questions. It helped tremendously!

Kami Jackson and Amy Waters: Thank you for creating Living Well and inviting me to be part of the team. Your vision of holistic mental wellness is revolutionary. You are both safe spaces to so many, including me.

The entire Living Well team: Every single one of you inspired pieces of this book. Thank you to the massage therapists who calm my nervous system with touch, the yoga teachers who balance my breathing, the guest relations team who patiently listen to me ramble, and the therapists who remind me of the roles attachment theory, trauma, and internal family systems play in our holistic design. You all inspire me daily.

ACKNOWLEDGMENTS

Katharine Elkins: First, I am grateful for your loyal friendship. Thank you for connecting me to Denison Forum and encouraging me to keep writing (and also for taking pictures of my good side).

Denison Forum: Thank you for allowing me to share about the nuances of faith and mental health.

My friends: Amanda Hyman and Amanda Weaver, you read the very early edition of this manuscript, and your feedback propelled me forward in hopes that I was onto something. Lindsay Berryman, thank you for always helping me think outside the box. Hannah Estes and Amber Herrin, thank you for the decades of friendship and reminders that I need to have fun too. Elise Carter, thank you for all the walks and neurodivergent rabbit trails that inspired so much of this writing process. Amber Volbeda and Linda Arnold, if not for you two, I wouldn't have taken the dive into learning about gut health. Thank you for supporting me.

My English teachers, who encouraged me to write: We did it! Mrs. Silvera (second grade), you gave me hope and told me my name would be on a book one day. Mrs. Barbara Johnson (middle school), you taught me structure and the importance of transitions. Ms. Marianne Bowers (high school), you saw through my "happy" mask and encouraged me that my name would be on a book cover. Dr. Catherine Ross (undergraduate English studies), you taught me the power of using nature walks for inspiration, as our buddy Wordsworth did.

Janet Taylor, my high school science teacher: You recently reminded me that I declared, "I'll never use this stuff," referring to everything you taught me in class. Yep, the joke's on me. All the citations are for you. Turns out, cells really are relevant.

Tracy Harrison, founder and lead educator of the School of Applied Functional Medicine: Your training completely changed my coaching methods and helped me appreciate the interconnectedness of all things.

Millie Tanner, my therapist: Thank you for (still) reminding me that I actually don't have to analyze my feelings. I can just feel them.

Our Sunday night small group crew—the Weavers, Beardens, Rosses, Denmons, Youngs, and Bumgardners: Thank you for your prayers and for allowing me to share during this book writing process.

My clients, past and present: Thank you for trusting me with your stories and for letting me help you put the puzzle pieces together.

Finally, to God: Your three-in-one being is instrumental in my understanding about the intelligent design of my body, mind, and spirit. That design has inspired over a decade of study on how to integrate wholeness into my life and the lives of others. It is your Spirit who reminds me that my Big Feelings are safe with you, always. It is your Son who reminds me it's okay to express those feelings. Thank you for showing me I'm not alone.

Notes

THE LABELS WE WEAR

1. "Mental Health Disorder Statistics," Johns Hopkins Medicine, n.d., https://www.hopkinsmedicine.org/health/wellness-and-prevention/mental-health-disorder-statistics.
2. Peter Boersma, Lindsey I. Black, and Brian W. Ward, "Prevalence of Multiple Chronic Conditions among US Adults, 2018," *Preventing Chronic Disease* 17 (September 17, 2020): 1–4, e106, https://doi.org/10.5888/pcd17.200130.
3. Lissa Rankin, MD, *Mind over Medicine: Scientific Proof That You Can Heal Yourself* (Carlsbad, CA: Hay House, 2013), 34.
4. "Functional Medicine vs. Lifestyle Medicine," Peak Integrative Medicine, n.d., https://peakintegrativemed.com/functional-medicine-vs-lifestyle-medicine.

CHAPTER 1: AN INVITATION TO EXAMINE THE LABEL

1. In reference to mental health, *hypervigilance* describes a brain that is constantly alert and scanning for threats. It is a protective state activated for survival and is often the result of trauma.
2. *The Diagnostic and Statistical Manual of Mental Disorders* is the reference manual used by practitioners to diagnose mental disorders. Often referred to by its acronym DSM-5-TR, it is currently on its fifth edition, which was published in 2022. Some critics believe it is overly subjective, which can lead to misdiagnosis and cause confusion for patients looking for clear answers to their issues.
3. Gabor Maté, *The Myth of Normal: Trauma, Illness, and Healing in a Toxic Culture* (New York: Avery, 2022), 16.

4. Dr. Caroline Leaf, *Cleaning Up Your Mental Mess: Five Simple, Scientifically Proven Steps to Reduce Anxiety, Stress, and Toxic Thinking* (Grand Rapids: Baker Books, 2021), 158.
5. Leaf, *Cleaning Up Your Mental Mess*, 74.

CHAPTER 2: THE TWO TYPES OF STRESS DRAINING US ALL

1. Stress is so common today that one study estimated up to 90 percent of chronic disease is stress related. See Yun-Zi Liu, Yun-Xia Wang, and Chun-Lei Jiang, "Inflammation: The Common Pathway of Stress-Related Diseases," *Frontiers in Human Neuroscience* 11 (June 20, 2017): 316, https://doi.org/10.3389/fnhum.2017.00316.
2. "Stress," Cleveland Clinic, n.d., https://my.clevelandclinic.org/health/diseases/11874-stress.
3. Jeffrey D. Galley et al., "Exposure to a Social Stressor Disrupts the Community Structure of the Colonic Mucosa-Associated Microbiota," *BMC Microbiology* 14, no. 189 (July 15, 2014), https://doi.org/10.1186/1471-2180-14-189.
4. Julia Ross, *The Mood Cure: The Four-Step Program to Take Charge of Your Emotions—Today* (New York: Penguin, 2004), 93.
5. "The Link Between Contraceptive Pills and Depression," *Neuroscience News*, June 13, 2023, https://neurosciencenews.com/depression-contraceptive-pills-23451.
6. Maria Godoy, "What We Know about the Health Risks of Ultra-Processed Foods," *All Things Considered*, NPR, May 25, 2023, https://www.npr.org/sections/health-shots/2023/05/25/1178163270/ultra-processed-foods-health-risk-weight-gain.
7. One research study even claimed that Oreo cookies are more addictive than cocaine! George Dvorsky, "How 'Hyperpalatable' Foods Could Turn You into a Food Addict," *Gizmodo*, May 12, 2014, https://gizmodo.com/how-hyperpalatable-foods-could-turn-you-into-a-food-add-1575144399.
8. Victoria J. Drake, "Micronutrient Inadequacies in the US Population: An Overview," Oregon State University, November 2017, https://lpi.oregonstate.edu/mic/micronutrient-inadequacies/overview.
9. Georgia Ede, MD, *Change Your Diet, Change Your Mind: A Powerful Plan to Improve Mood, Overcome Anxiety, and Protect Memory for a Lifetime of Optimal Mental Health* (New York: Balance, 2024), 108.
10. Kendra Cherry, "What Is Allostatic Load?," Verywell Mind, updated August 11, 2022, https://www.verywellmind.com/what-is-allostatic-load-5680283.
11. Oxford Languages, s.v. "nourishment," https://bit.ly/3LLCNiw.
12. This idea is closely connected to the concept of "primary food," a term coined by Joshua Rosenthal, founder and director of the Institute for

NOTES

Integrative Nutrition, which I attended. For more, see Joshua Rosenthal, *The Power of Primary Food: Tools for Nourishment Beyond the Plate* (New York: Integrative Nutrition Publishing, 2015).

CHAPTER 3: HOW YOUR SELF-TALK IMPACTS YOUR HEALTH

1. Secretory immunoglobulin A is the first line of defense in the intestines, playing an essential role in the mucosal barrier to protect against pathogens and prevent infections in the immune system. N. J. Mantis, N. Rol, and B. Corthésy, "Secretory IgA's Complex Roles in Immunity and Mucosal Homeostasis in the Gut," *Mucosal Immunology* 4, no. 6 (October 5, 2011): 603–611, https://doi.org/10.1038/mi.2011.41.
2. Glen Rein, Mike Atkinson, and Rollin McCraty, "The Physiological and Psychological Effects of Compassion and Anger," *Journal of Advancement in Medicine* 8, no. 2 (1995): 87–105, https://www.heartmath.org/assets/uploads/2015/01/compassion-and-anger.pdf.
3. Bruce H. Lipton, PhD, *The Biology of Belief: Unleashing the Power of Consciousness, Matter, and Miracles* (Carlsbad, CA: Hay House, 2016), 139.
4. "Hypothalamic-Pituitary-Adrenal (HPA) Axis," Cleveland Clinic, April 12, 2024, https://my.clevelandclinic.org/health/body/hypothalamic-pituitary-adrenal-hpa-axis.
5. Dr. Wendy Suzuki with Billie Fitzpatrick, *Good Anxiety: Harnessing the Power of the Most Misunderstood Emotion* (New York: Atria Books, 2021), 44.
6. *APA Dictionary of Psychology*, s.v. "trait negativity bias," American Psychological Association, updated April 19, 2018, https://dictionary.apa.org/trait-negativity-bias.
7. Bessel van der Kolk, MD, *The Body Keeps the Score: Brain, Mind, and Body in the Healing of Trauma* (New York: Penguin Books, 2015), 55.
8. Terrence Deak et al., "Neuroimmune Mechanisms of Stress: Sex Differences, Developmental Plasticity, and Implications for Pharmacotherapy of Stress-Related Disease," *Stress* 18, no. 4 (July 2015): 367–380, https://doi.org/10.3109/10253890.2015.1053451.
9. Ellen Doney et al., "Inflammation-Driven Brain and Gut Barrier Dysfunction in Stress and Mood Disorders," *European Journal of Neuroscience* 55, no. 9–10 (May 2022): 2851–2894, https://doi.org/10.1111/ejn.15239.
10. Donna Jackson Nakazawa, *The Angel and the Assassin: The Tiny Brain Cell That Changed the Course of Medicine* (New York: Ballantine Books, 2020), 93.
11. Rein, Atkinson, and McCraty, "The Physiological and Psychological Effects."
12. Adrienne A. Taren, J. David Creswell, and Peter J. Gianaros, "Dispositional Mindfulness Co-Varies with Smaller Amygdala and Caudate Volumes in Community Adults," *PLOS ONE* 8, no. 5 (May 22, 2013): e64574, https://doi.org/10.1371/journal.pone.0064574.

13. This saying is a summary of Donald Hebb's 1949 pioneering theory in the field of synaptic plasticity and memory. See Dong Il Choi and Bong-Kiun Kaang, "Interrogating Structural Plasticity Among Synaptic Engrams," *Current Opinion in Neurobiology* 75 (May 2022), https://doi.org/10.1016/j.conb.2022.102552.

CHAPTER 4: COULD YOUR PESKY THOUGHTS BE PROTECTIVE?

1. Jennifer Tucker, *Breath as Prayer: Calm Your Anxiety, Focus Your Mind, and Renew Your Soul* (Nashville: Thomas Nelson, 2022), 50–51.

CHAPTER 5: YOUR BREATH REFLECTS YOUR STRESS LEVELS

1. Dr. Andrew Weil, quoted in James Nestor, *Breath: The New Science of a Lost Art* (New York: Riverhead Books, 2020), 206.
2. Nestor, *Breath*, 55.
3. "Breathwork Protocols for Health, Focus and Stress," Huberman Lab, October 6, 2023, https://www.hubermanlab.com/newsletter/breathwork-protocols-for-health-focus-stress.
4. Gunjan Y. Trivedi et al., "Humming (Simple Bhramari Pranayama) as a Stress Buster: A Holter-Based Study to Analyze Heart Rate Variability (HRV) Parameters During Bhramari, Physical Activity, Emotional Stress, and Sleep," *Cureus* 15, no. 4 (April 13, 2023): e37527, https://doi.org/10.7759/cureus.37527.
5. Shirley Telles et al., "Alternate-Nostril Yoga Breathing Reduced Blood Pressure While Increasing Performance in a Vigilance Test," *Medical Science Monitor Basic Research* 23 (December 2017): 392–398, https://doi.org/10.12659/msmbr.906502.

CHAPTER 6: IS IT ME OR MY TRAUMA RESPONSE?

1. Although PTSD is sometimes used interchangeably with CPTSD (complex post-traumatic stress disorder), they are different. While PTSD is caused by a single traumatic event, CPTSD is caused by ongoing trauma that lasts for months or years.
2. "Traumatic Memories Are Represented Differently than Regular Sad Memories in the Brains of People with PTSD, New Research Shows," press release, Mount Sinai, November 30, 2023, https://www.mountsinai.org/about/newsroom/2023/traumatic-memories-are-represented-differently-than-regular-sad-memories-in-the-brains-of-people-with-ptsd-new-research-shows.
3. Hypersensitivity is not to be confused with the term *Highly Sensitive Person (HSP)*, a neurodivergent individual who processes emotions differently and has a heightened response to stimuli. However, being an HSP does make recovering from trauma more difficult.

NOTES

4. "Eye Movement Desensitization and Reprocessing (EMDR) is a psychotherapy treatment that is designed to alleviate the distress associated with traumatic memories." See "What Is EMDR Therapy?," EMDR Institute, https://www.emdr.com/what-is-emdr.
5. Melissa T. Merrick et al., "Vital Signs: Estimated Proportion of Adult Health Problems Attributable to Adverse Childhood Experiences and Implications for Prevention—25 States, 2015–2017," *Morbidity and Mortality Weekly Report* 68, no. 44 (November 8, 2019): 999–1005, https://doi.org/10.15585/mmwr.mm6844e1.
6. Sara Szal Gottfried, MD, *The Autoimmune Cure: Healing the Trauma and Other Triggers That Have Turned Your Body Against You* (New York: Harvest, 2024), 27.
7. Ali Jawaid, Martin Roszkowski, and Isabelle M. Mansuy, "Chapter Twelve: Transgenerational Epigenetics of Traumatic Stress," *Progress in Molecular Biology and Translational Science* 158 (2018): 273–298, https://www.sciencedirect.com/science/article/abs/pii/S187711731830053X?via%3Dihub.
8. Rachel Yehuda et al., "Gene Expression Patterns Associated with Posttraumatic Stress Disorder Following Exposure to the World Trade Center Attacks" *Biological Psychiatry* 66, no. 7 (April 27, 2009): 708–711, https://doi.org/10.1016/j.biopsych.2009.02.034.
9. *APA Dictionary of Psychology*, s.v. "grief," American Psychological Association, updated April 19, 2018, https://dictionary.apa.org/grief.

CHAPTER 7: THE COPING MECHANISMS THAT KEPT YOU SAFE

1. Eline Feenstra, "Dopamine Plays Double Duty in Learning and Motivation," *Neuroscience News*, June 6, 2023, https://neurosciencenews.com/dopamine-motivation-learning-23403.
2. Tamara Rosier, PhD, *Your Brain's Not Broken: Strategies for Navigating Your Emotions and Life with ADHD* (Grand Rapids: Revell, 2021), 56.

CHAPTER 8: UNBLOCKING YOUR FEELINGS

1. Karla McLaren, "Is It a Feeling or Is It an Emotion?," karlacclaren.com, March 3, 2012, https://karlamclaren.com/is-it-a-feeling-or-is-it-an-emotion-revisited.
2. Gloria Willcox, "The Feeling Wheel: A Tool for Expanding Awareness of Emotions and Increasing Spontaneity and Intimacy," *Transactional Analysis Journal* 12, no. 4 (October 1982): 274–276, https://doi.org/10.1177/036215378201200411.
3. Gloria Willcox, "The Feeling Wheel," All the Feelz, n.d., https://allthefeelz.app/feeling-wheel. Licensed under a Creative Commons Attribution-ShareAlike 4.0 International License, https://creativecommons.org/licenses/by-sa/4.0.

CHAPTER 9: LOOKING FOR A MAGIC FIX

1. The MTHFR gene provides instructions for making an enzyme called methylenetetrahydrofolate reductase, which is important for a chemical reaction involving the vitamin folate, vitamin B9. Improving expression of this gene is far more complicated than simply eliminating folic acid, but it is often given a lot of attention in groups that focus on holistic health, which can cause confusion and distress.
2. Autoimmune diseases occur when the immune system, out of protection, becomes overactive and targets its own healthy cells, tissues, and organs. There are over eighty different types of autoimmune diseases. Studies show that 25 percent of people who are diagnosed with one autoimmune disease will at some point be diagnosed with another. Manole Cojocaru, Inimioara Mihaela Cojocaru, and Isabela Silosi, "Multiple Autoimmune Syndrome," *Maedica* 5, no. 2 (April 2010): 132–134, https://www.ncbi.nlm.nih.gov/pmc/articles/PMC3150011.

CHAPTER 10: A BODY IN STRESS WON'T DIGEST

1. Wolfgang Langhans, Alan G. Watts, and Alan C. Spector, "The Elusive Cephalic Phase Insulin Response: Triggers, Mechanisms, and Functions," *Physiological Reviews* 103, no. 2 (February 15, 2023): 1423–1485, https://doi.org/10.1152/physrev.00025.2022.
2. Alia J. Crum et al., "Mind over Milkshakes: Mindsets, Not Just Nutrients, Determine Ghrelin Response," *Health Psychology* 30, no. 4 (July 2011): 424–429, discussion 430–431, https://pubmed.ncbi.nlm.nih.gov/21574706.

CHAPTER 11: USING FOOD TO SUPPORT YOUR MOOD

1. MSG stands for monosodium glutamate, which is a flavor enhancer in most processed foods. It gives food that irresistible, "can't-put-it-down" quality.
2. Yusuke Hirata, "Trans-Fatty Acids as an Enhancer of Inflammation and Cell Death: Molecular Basis for Their Pathological Actions," *Biological and Pharmaceutical Bulletin* 44, no. 10 (2021): 1349–1356, https://www.jstage.jst.go.jp/article/bpb/44/10/44_b21-00449/_article.
3. Arne Astrup et al., "Saturated Fats and Health: A Reassessment and Proposal for Food-Based Recommendations," *Journal of the American College of Cardiology* 76, no. 7 (August 2020): 844–857, https://doi.org/10.1016/j.jacc.2020.05.077.
4. Georgia Ede, MD, *Change Your Diet, Change Your Mind: A Powerful Plan to Improve Mood, Overcome Anxiety, and Protect Memory for a Lifetime of Optimal Mental Health* (New York: Balance, 2024), 61.
5. Erin P. Ferranti et al., "Twenty Things You Didn't Know about the Human Gut Microbiome," *Journal of Cardiovascular Nursing* 29, no. 6

NOTES

(November/December 2014): 479–481, https://doi.org/10.1097/jcn.0000000000000166.

6. Leo Galland, "The Gut Microbiome and the Brain," *Journal of Medicine and Food* 17, no. 12 (December 2014): 1261–1272, https://pubmed.ncbi.nlm.nih.gov/25402818.
7. Dinyadarshini Johnson et al., "A Microbial-Based Approach to Mental Health: The Potential of Probiotics in the Treatment of Depression," *Nutrients* 15, no. 6 (March 13, 2023): 1382, https://www.mdpi.com/2072-6643/15/6/1382.
8. "Lashing Out at Your Spouse? Check Your Blood Sugar," Ohio State University, April 14, 2014, https://news.osu.edu/lashing-out-at-your-spouse-check-your-blood-sugar.
9. David S. Ludwig et al., "High Glycemic Index Foods, Overeating, and Obesity," *Pediatrics* 103, no. 3 (March 1, 1999): e26, https://doi.org/10.1542/peds.103.3.e26.
10. Bruce Goldman, "Insulin Resistance Doubles Risk of Major Depressive Disorder, Stanford Study Finds," Stanford Medicine News Center, September 22, 2021, https://med.stanford.edu/news/all-news/2021/09/insulin-resistance-major-depressive-disorder.html.
11. Erin Kerry, host, *Sparking Wholeness,* podcast, episode 180, "The Missing Puzzle Piece to Your Mental Health Struggles with Rachael Bevilacqua and Dr. Kate Kresge (Kate Henry)," April 3, 2023, https://www.toginet.com/podcasts/sparkingwholeness/SparkingWholenessLIVE_2023_04_03.mp3?type=podpage.
12. Hideaki Sato et al., "Protein Deficiency-Induced Behavioral Abnormalities and Neurotransmitter Loss in Aged Mice Are Ameliorated by Essential Amino Acids," *Frontiers in Nutrition* 7 (March 2020), https://doi.org/10.3389/fnut.2020.00023.
13. Laura R. LaChance and Drew Ramsey, "Antidepressant Foods: An Evidence-Based Nutrient Profiling System for Depression," *World Journal of Psychiatry* 8, no. 3 (September 20, 2018): 97–104, https://pubmed.ncbi.nlm.nih.gov/30254980.
14. Drew Ramsey, MD, *Eat to Beat Depression and Anxiety: Nourish Your Way to Better Mental Health in Six Weeks* (New York: HarperCollins, 2021), 24.
15. Paola Bressan and Peter Kramer, "Bread and Other Edible Agents of Mental Disease," *Frontiers in Human Neuroscience* 10 (March 28, 2016), https://doi.org/10.3389/fnhum.2016.00130.
16. Alessio Fasano, "All Disease Begins in the (Leaky) Gut: Role of Zonulin-Mediated Gut Permeability in the Pathogenesis of Some Chronic Inflammatory Diseases," *F1000Research* 9, no. 1 (January 31, 2020): 69, https://doi.org/10.12688/f1000research.20510.1.
17. Anthony Samsel and Stephanie Seneff, "Glyphosate, Pathways to Modern Diseases II: Celiac Sprue and Gluten Intolerance," *Interdisciplinary*

Toxicology 6, no. 4 (December 2013): 159–184, https://doi.org/10.2478/intox-2013-0026.

CHAPTER 12: WEIGHT ISSUES AND RESTORING BODY PEACE

1. Jen Carter, PhD, "That Diet Probably Won't Work Long-Term—Here's What to Focus on Instead," Ohio State Health and Discovery, February 1, 2022, https://health.osu.edu/wellness/exercise-and-nutrition/that-diet-probably-did-not-work.
2. Chika Anekwe, MD, MPH, "Exercise, Metabolism, and Weight: New Research from *The Biggest Loser*," Harvard Health Publishing, January 27, 2022, https://www.health.harvard.edu/blog/exercise-metabolism-and-weight-new-research-from-the-biggest-loser-202201272676#:~:text=Taken%20together%2C%20what%20we.
3. Peter Sjöstedt, Jesper Enander, and Josef Isung, "Serotonin Reuptake Inhibitors and the Gut Microbiome: Significance of the Gut Microbiome in Relation to Mechanism of Action, Treatment Response, Side Effects, and Tachyphylaxis," *Frontiers in Psychiatry* 12 (May 25, 2021), https://doi.org/10.3389/fpsyt.2021.682868.
4. Maurizio Fava, "Weight Gain and Antidepressants," *Journal of Clinical Psychiatry* 61, supplement 11 (September 30, 2000): 37–41, https://pubmed.ncbi.nlm.nih.gov/10926053/.
5. Christopher M. Palmer, MD, *Brain Energy: A Revolutionary Breakthrough in Understanding Mental Health—and Improving Treatment for Anxiety, Depression, OCD, PTSD, and More* (Dallas: BenBella Books, 2022), 191.
6. Brooks R. Keeshin et al., "Sexual Abuse Is Associated with Obese Children and Adolescents Admitted for Psychiatric Hospitalization," *Journal of Pediatrics* 163, no. 1 (July 2013): 154–159, https://pubmed.ncbi.nlm.nih.gov/23414663/.
7. Xiaoya Guo et al., "Pro-Inflammatory Immunological Effects of Adipose Tissue and Risk of Food Allergy in Obesity: Focus on Immunological Mechanisms," *Allergologia et Immunopathologia* 48, no. 3 (May-June 2020): 306–312, https://www.sciencedirect.com/science/article/abs/pii/S0301054619300904?via%3Dihub.
8. Erin Jackson et al., "Adipose Tissue as a Site of Toxin Accumulation," *Comprehensive Physiology* 7, no. 4 (September 12, 2017): 1085–1135, https://pubmed.ncbi.nlm.nih.gov/28915320/.
9. Ronald Hoffman, MD, "Ultra-Processed Food Consumption, Appetite, and Weight Gain," *Natural Medicine Journal*, July 2, 2019, https://www.naturalmedicinejournal.com/journal/ultra-processed-food-consumption-appetite-and-weight-gain.
10. Linda Bacon, *Health at Every Size: The Surprising Truth about Your Weight* (Dallas, TX: Benbella Books, 2010), 267.
11. Alice Chirico and Andrea Gaggioli, "The Potential Role of Awe for

NOTES

Depression: Reassembling the Puzzle," *Frontiers in Psychology* 12 (April 26, 2021), https://doi.org/10.3389/fpsyg.2021.617715.

12. Christine Valters Paintner, *The Wisdom of the Body: A Contemplative Journey to Wholeness for Women* (Notre Dame, IN: Sorin Books, 2017), 190.

PART 4: EXERCISE YOUR BODY AND BRAIN

1. Darren Hardy, *The Compound Effect: Jumpstart Your Income, Your Life, Your Success* (New York: Hachette, 2020), 13.

CHAPTER 13: ENGAGING IN HEALTHY EMOTIONAL REGULATION

1. Bessel van der Kolk, *The Body Keeps the Score: Brain, Mind, and Body in the Healing of Trauma* (New York: Penguin Books, 2015), 99.
2. Robby Berman, "Having a Sense of Purpose May Help You Live Longer, Research Shows," *MedicalNewsToday*, November 21, 2022, https://www.medicalnewstoday.com/articles/longevity-having-a-purpose-may-help-you-live-longer-healthier.
3. *NIV Exhaustive Concordance Dictionary*, accessed on Bible Gateway Plus, https://www.biblegateway.com/passage/?search=john%2015%3A4&version=NIV.
4. David Perlmutter, MD, and Austin Perlmutter, MD, *Brain Wash: Detox Your Mind for Clearer Thinking, Deeper Relationships, and Lasting Happiness* (New York: Little, Brown and Company, 2020), 43.

CHAPTER 14: MOVEMENT AS MEDICINE

1. John J. Ratey, MD, with Eric Hagerman, *Spark: The Revolutionary New Science of Exercise and the Brain* (New York: Little, Brown and Company, 2008), 45.
2. Wei Chen et al., "Aerobic Exercise Improves Food Reward Systems in Obese Rats via Insulin Signaling Regulation of Dopamine Levels in the Nucleus Accumbens," *ACS Chemical Neuroscience* 10, no. 6 (April 22, 2019): 2801–2808, https://doi.org/10.1021/acschemneuro.9b00022.
3. Ben Singh et al., "Effectiveness of Physical Activity Interventions for Improving Depression, Anxiety and Distress: An Overview of Systematic Reviews," *British Journal of Sports Medicine* 57, no. 18 (September 2023): 1203–1209, https://doi.org/10.1136/bjsports-2022-106195.
4. Devi Sridhar, "The Secret to Why Exercise Is So Good for Mental Health? 'Hope Molecules,'" *Guardian*, May 4, 2023, https://www.theguardian.com/commentisfree/2023/may/04/exercise-mental-health-hope-molecules-mood-strength.
5. "The More You Walk, the Lower Your Risk of Early Death, Even If You Walk Fewer than 5,000 Steps," *Science Daily*, August 8, 2023, https://www.sciencedaily.com/releases/2023/08/230808201935.htm.

CHAPTER 15: HEALING THROUGH REST

1. "Burn-Out an 'Occupational Phenomenon,'" World Health Organization, https://www.who.int/standards/classifications/frequently-asked-questions/burn-out-an-occupational-phenomenon.
2. "*QuickStats:* Percentage of Adults Aged ≥18 Years Who Sleep <7 Hours on Average in a 24-Hour Period, by Sex and Age Group—National Health Interview Survey, United States, 2020," *Morbidity and Mortality Weekly Report* 71, no. 10 (March 11, 2022): 393, https://doi.org/10.15585/mmwr.mm7110a6.
3. Dzifa Adjaye-Gbewonyo, Amanda E. Ng, and Lindsey I. Black, "Sleep Difficulties in Adults: United States, 2020," *NCHS Data Brief*, no. 436 (June 2022), https://www.cdc.gov/nchs/data/databriefs/db436.pdf. See also "Sleep Statistics and Facts," National Council on Aging, March 7, 2024, https://www.ncoa.org/adviser/sleep/sleep-statistics.
4. Andrew Huberman, "Using Light for Health," Huberman Lab, Neural Network Newsletter, January 24, 2023, https://www.hubermanlab.com/newsletter/using-light-for-health.
5. Matthew Walker, *Why We Sleep: Unlocking the Power of Sleep and Dreams* (New York: Scribner, 2017), 27.
6. Pia Christ et al., "The Circadian Clock Drives Mast Cell Functions in Allergic Reactions," *Frontiers in Immunology* 9 (July 6, 2018), https://doi.org/10.3389/fimmu.2018.01526.
7. Walker, *Why We Sleep*, 275.
8. To learn more about NSDR, which is also known as yoga nidra, see, Jay Summer and Dr. Brandon Peters, "What Is Non-Sleep Deep Rest (NSDR)?" Sleep Foundation, February 26, 2024, https://www.sleepfoundation.org/meditation-for-sleep/what-is-non-sleep-deep-rest.

About the Author

Erin Kerry is an integrative health coach and functional nutritionist. She is the host of the top-ranked podcast *Sparking Wholeness* and the owner of the coaching company Sparking Wholeness.

As a survivor of mental illness, Erin knows firsthand how suffering from a chronic illness can infiltrate every area of life. By the age of eighteen, she was given the labels PTSD, depression, and bipolar disorder. She became pregnant at twenty-two, after a very self-destructive phase of her mental health journey, marked by mania, alcohol, and poor medication management. Today, she is living beyond her labels and is symptom-free. Through her story and her integrative nutrition training, Erin empowers others to be their own health advocates so they don't have to be limited by a label or diagnosis.

She is a regular contributor to online publications on the topic of mental health and wellness. Aside from coaching hundreds of individuals, she frequently speaks to groups and businesses.

She and her pastor-turned-counselor husband, Richard, both work at Living Well Holistic Counseling and Wellness Center in Tyler, Texas. They have three children: Isabel, Roman, and Rhett. Erin's favorite nonwork activities are reading fiction, playing games with her family, watching her kids play sports and music, making (and eating) nutrient-dense food, taking nature walks, practicing yoga, and traveling anywhere—when she can!